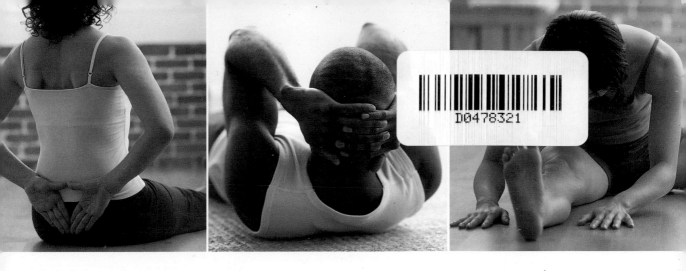

The Body Shop

Yoga

Aurum Press

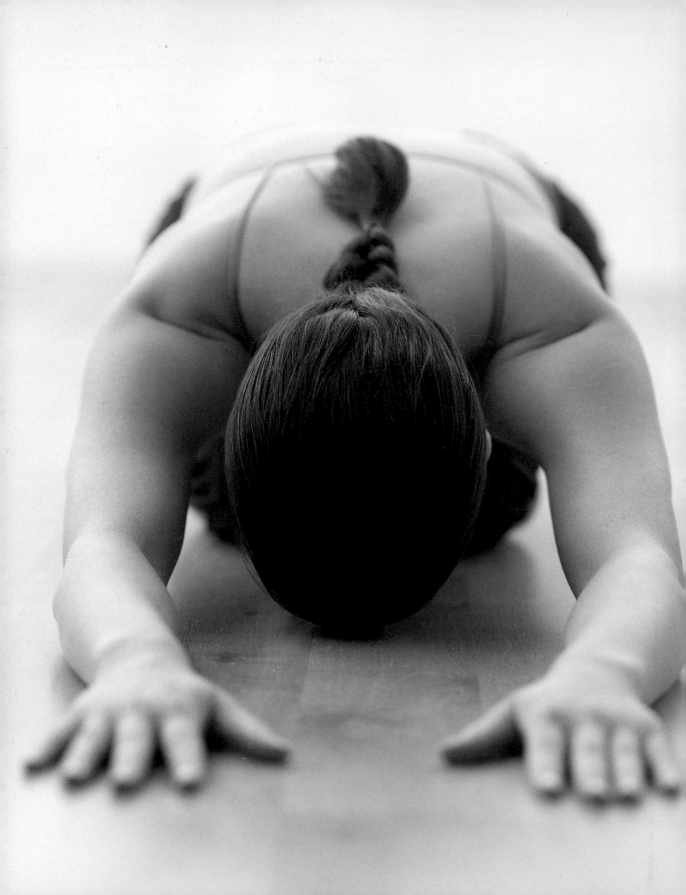

The Body Shop

Yoga

kristie dahlia home

photography by john robbins

First Published in Great Britain
2005 by Aurum Press Ltd
25 Bedford Avenue, London WC1B 3AT

THE BODY SHOP INTERNATIONAL, PLC
Founder, Non-Executive Director Dame Anita Roddick
Chairman Adrian Bellamy
Chief Executive Officer Peter Saunders
Director of Product Paul McGreevy
Publications Manager Justine Roddick

WELDON OWEN INC.
Chief Executive Officer John Owen
Chief Operating Officer and President Terry Newell
Vice President and Publisher Roger Shaw
Vice President, International Sales Stuart Laurence

Publisher Rebecca Poole Forée
Creative Director Gaye Allen
Senior Art Director Emma Boys
Art Director Colin Wheatland
Managing Editor Elizabeth Dougherty
Production Director Chris Hemesath
Colour Manager Teri Bell
Co-Edition and Reprint Coordinator Todd Rechner
Designers Rachel Lopez, Adrienne Aquino
Consulting Editor Maria Behan
Anglicization Grant Laing Partnership

The Body Shop Yoga was conceived and produced by Weldon Owen Inc., 814 Montgomery Street, San Francisco, California 94133, United States, in collaboration with The Body Shop International PLC, Watersmead, Littlehampton, West Sussex, BN17 6LS, United Kingdom. The Body Shop™ trademark application pending.

A WELDON OWEN PRODUCTION
Copyright © 2005 Weldon Owen Inc.
All rights reserved, including the right of reproduction in whole or in part in any form.

Set in Bembo™ and Benton Gothic™
Colour separations by Bright Arts, Hong Kong
Printed in China by Midas Printing Limited

10 9 8 7 6 5 4 3 2
2008 2007 2006 2005

A catalogue record for this book is available from the British Library.

ISBN 1-84513-077-4

A NOTE ABOUT THIS BOOK
This book was printed using soy-based inks on Forest Stewardship Council–approved paper. The book is bound with non-toxic glue made from non-animal sources..

DISCLAIMER
This book is not intended as a medical reference guide. The advice contained herein is not to be construed as medical diagnosis or treatment, and should not be used as a substitute for the advice of qualified health practitioners. Neither The Body Shop International, nor the publisher, nor the authors can be held responsible for adverse reactions, damage or injury resulting from the use of the content herein. Any application of yoga, aromatherapy or other suggestions that are contained herein is done at the reader's sole discretion and risk. During pregnancy or for serious or long-term problems, consult a health practitioner before using yoga or aromatherapy.

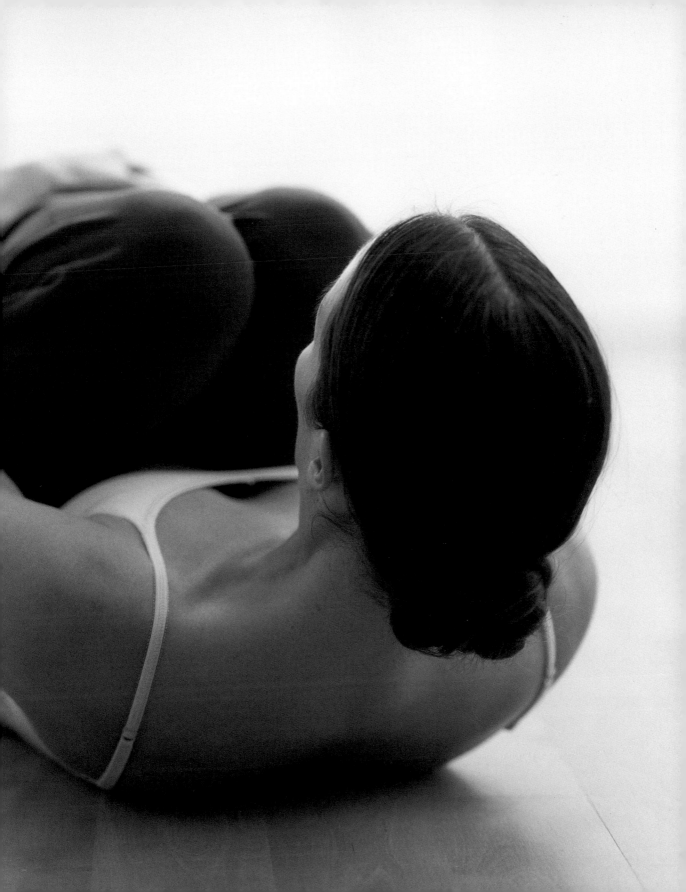

contents

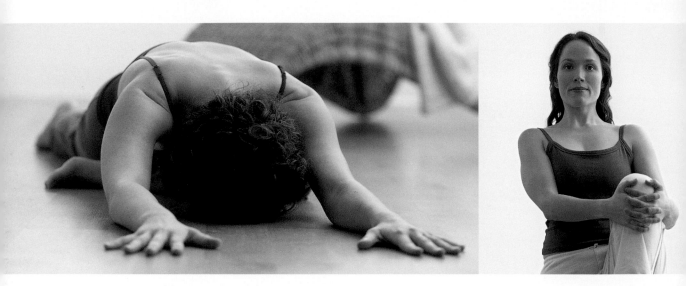

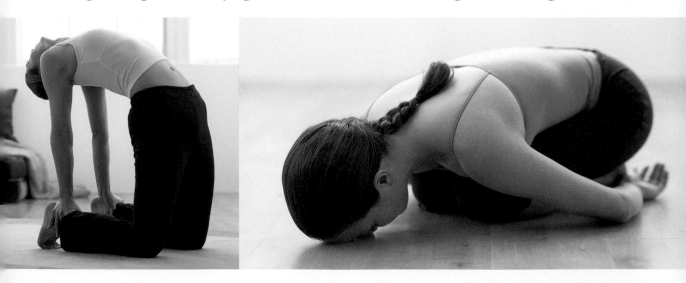

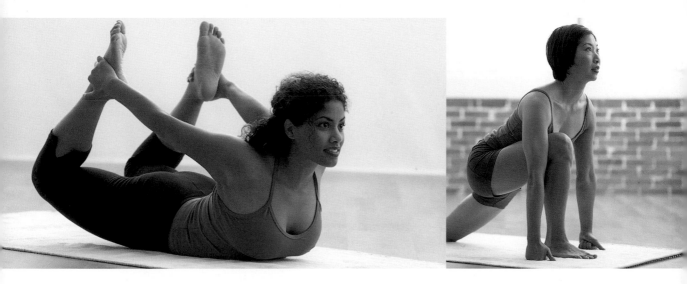

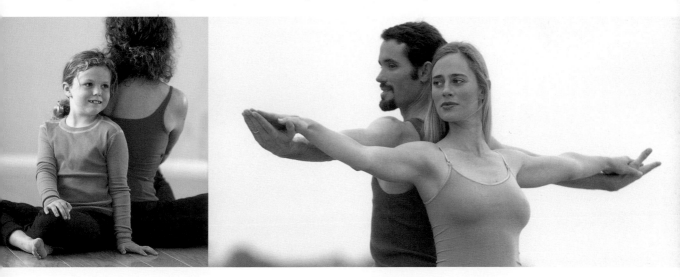

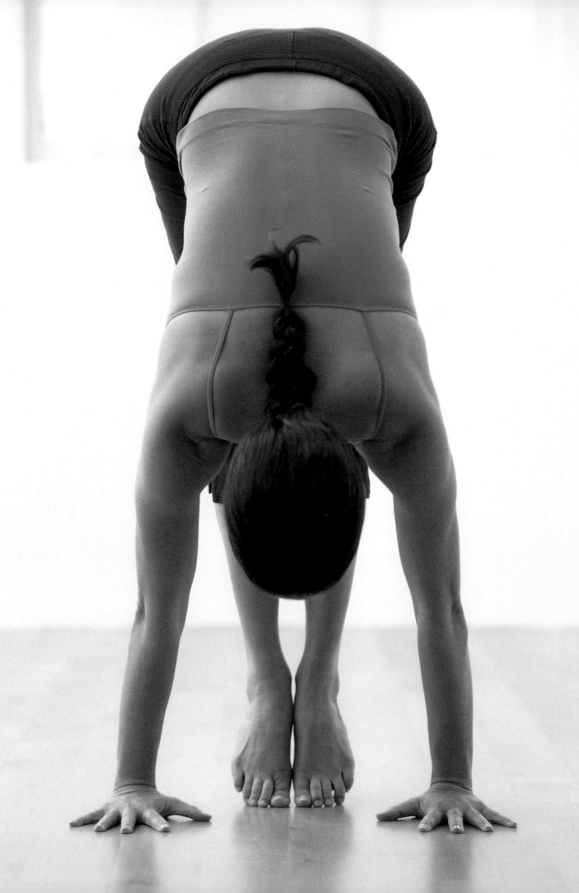

the gentle power of yoga

Yoga is a living tradition, an ancient Indian physical and mental system for self-exploration and growth. In Sanskrit, the word *yoga* means "union", from the root *yuj,* "to yoke or join together". Practising yoga harmonises, or "joins together", mind, body and spirit. Yoga's transformative power has been demonstrated over the centuries, and the latest scientific research attests to its many benefits.

Studies show that the practice of yoga can help increase cardiovascular and respiratory efficiency, aid in regulating endocrine and gastrointestinal function, and improve posture, strength, endurance and immunity. Research also shows that yoga offers benefits for mental health, such as improvements in mood, concentration and memory. When your body and mind function with clarity and efficiency, your natural wellbeing can shine through.

the basics of yoga practice

Yoga is more than mere stretching or exercise. It's a system for living that helps maximise health, serenity and happiness. It consists of a combination of *asanas* (poses), *pranayama* (breathing practices), and meditation. Yoga is a subtle, mindful activity; the finer aspects of how you work will determine the quality of your results. Stay conscious and be persistent; challenge yourself while also respecting your limits – and, most of all, enjoy your experience.

The sequences shown in this book are in the tradition of hatha yoga, a practice of asanas and pranayama that is currently undergoing a renaissance throughout the world. Derived from the Sanskrit words *ha* (sun) and *tha* (moon), hatha yoga strives to unite and balance the solar (energising) and lunar (relaxing) energies of the body. (Another branch of yoga, *raja* or "royal" yoga, includes a focus on meditation and the pursuit of ethical perfection. The spiritual concepts and meditative practices in this book originate in raja yoga.) Many yoga classes are offered in the hatha tradition, and you may want to find a class to complement your use of this book and help you establish an enjoyable ongoing practice.

defining your goals

The sequences in this book are designed so you can set your own goals. Some focus on strength or flexibility, others on mood or health. You may practise any sequence on its own. When you have more time, you may want to practise a full traditional cycle. Begin by warming up with the Sun Salutation (pages 16–17 ►), then practise a sequence or two of asanas (poses), and finally enjoy the deep relaxation described in Bliss (pages 108–111 ►). Follow with some breathing exercises (found throughout the book) and end with meditation (page 12 ►). A full cycle can last from 30 minutes to an hour or more. You might approach the same pose with a vigorous intent on one day and a calm one on another, with different physical and mental results. How you approach your practice affects the quality of your experience, so be aware of your mental state; try to clear your mind and harmonise your thinking with the result you are seeking, whether it's to calm, focus or energise.

asanas

An *asana* is a steady, comfortable yoga pose. This book is made up of groups of poses. Yoga practice develops the skills of effort and surrender and your ability to balance them. As you hold a pose, be sure you're not holding unnecessary tension in your body. Be as relaxed as possible while being precise.

You'll see that each asana has a suggested duration. Some durations are measured in breaths, and a breath equals one complete inhalation and exhalation. Please bear in mind that these hold times are suggestions: you may be comfortable holding a pose longer, or you may need to release it sooner. While holding a pose, observe your body; never push yourself into straining. Signals that you should release a pose are ragged breath, trembling or pain. Begin with short, easy hold times and gradually lengthen their duration with regular practice.

pranayama

In Sanskrit, *prana* means "life force" and *ayama* means "to increase". Yogic breathing exercises, called *pranayama,* are intended to increase our life force. You can practise pranayama on its own, during asanas or after yoga poses to calm, cleanse and invigorate. Physically, breathing nourishes on inhalation and cleanses

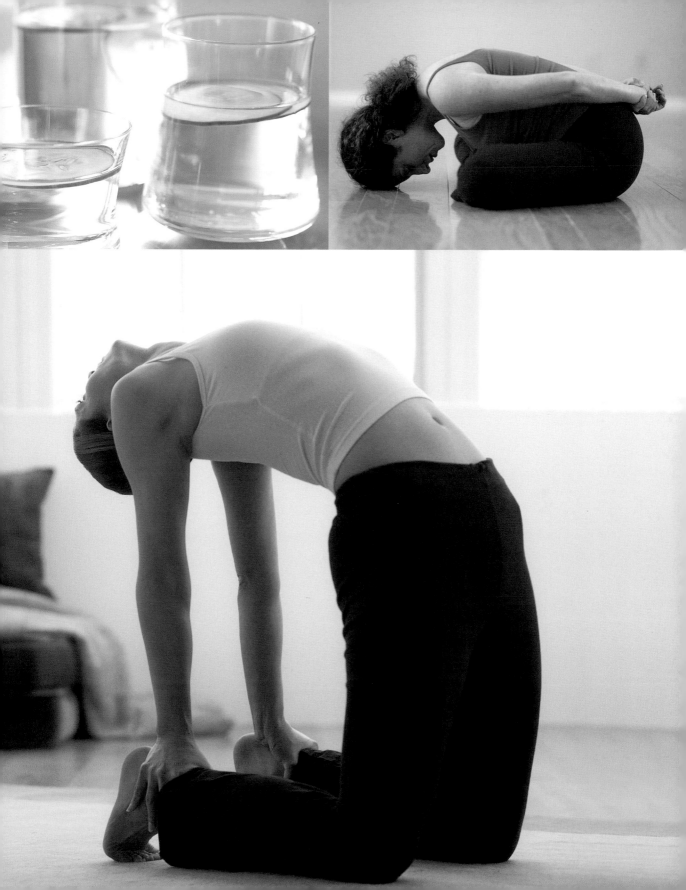

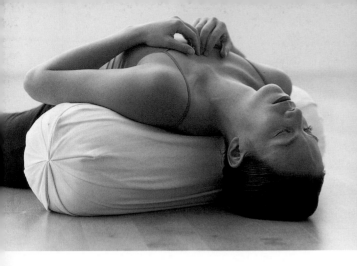
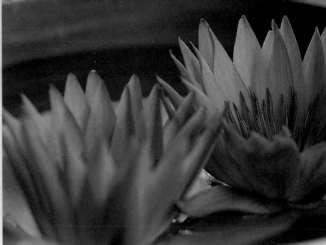

on exhalation. Practise pranayama on an empty stomach. Breathe through your nose and don't hold your breath unless otherwise instructed. If you feel light-headed, return to breathing normally. It's important to note that breath also is used in a deliberate way to help your body move into and out of poses. Inhalation is generally linked to movements that expand the chest or abdomen; exhalation is frequently linked to movements that compress the abdomen.

meditation

Meditation is a transformative state of consciousness that is approached by quieting the mind. This can seem difficult at first, since our minds tend to chatter, but the practice is simple. Just sit comfortably and try to focus your mind on one single thing. It's best to work with a consistent point of focus, such as your breath or a mantra. *Mantra japa* is the mental repetition of a word or phrase, traditionally linked to the pace of your breath. Repeating a mantra while holding a yoga pose can create a more meditative experience. You may use any uplifting phrase or word as a mantra, such as *shanti* (shahn-tee), which means "peace" in Sanskrit. If your mind wanders, simply draw it gently back to your point of focus. Try meditating for five minutes daily to start, increasing the duration over time.

heavenly scent

Aromatherapy is a centuries-old system of using fragrant essential oils distilled from plants to enhance mood and promote health. Essential oils can be diffused in the air during yoga practice, used in massage oils or dispersed in bath water, for example. Pure essential oils should almost never be applied undiluted directly on

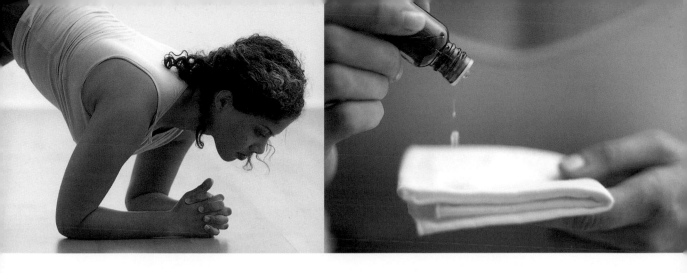

the skin. (Common carrier oils, used to dilute essential oils, include grapeseed, jojoba and sweet almond oil. Pre-blended aromatherapy oils are also available.) Always check the recommended amount and consult with an aromatherapist if you're unsure; if you are pregnant or have a medical condition, consult a doctor.

practising safely

Perform all movements gently, and stop at the very first sign of strain or pain (and try to learn to stop before you feel strain). When beginning any new programme of exercise, consult a doctor, especially if you are recovering from illness or injury. During pregnancy, your body and baby have unique needs that require the modification of your yoga practice. This book is not intended for pregnant women; if you are pregnant, seek out a specific prenatal yoga guide. Menstruation also calls for modifications to your practice (see Harmony, pages 70–75 ▶).

It's best to come to your yoga practice with an empty stomach (don't eat for at least two hours before) and wearing comfortable clothing. As with any exercise, it's important to drink plenty of water afterwards. It is traditional to practise with bare feet. A yoga mat adds comfort and helps prevent slipping.

Be sure to read the instructions for all the asanas in a sequence before you attempt them – don't just try to imitate the photographs. Properly entering into a pose can prevent injury, and some of the photos may show a more advanced version than you can comfortably hold. Remember that the quality of your efforts is more important than matching a pose in a photo. While holding poses, don't ever bounce; be steady and patient. A good rule of thumb is to work slowly and listen to your body. And if anything hurts, stop!

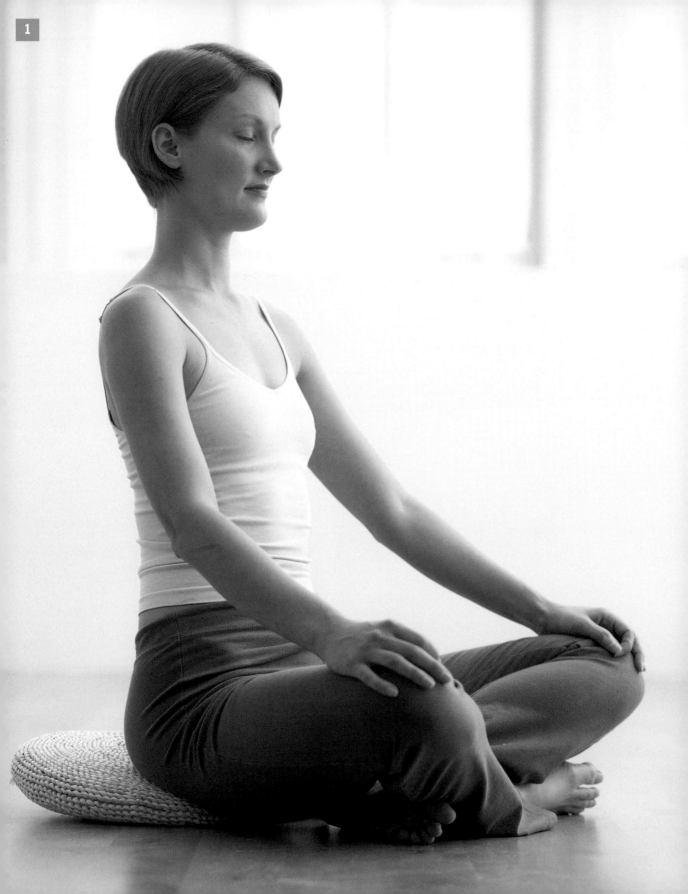

seated positions

When sitting for meditation or pranayama, focus on maintaining proper alignment, which requires (and builds) strength in your back and flexibility in your hips. If you feel discomfort, especially in your knees, find a more comfortable position or simply sit upright in a chair. Here are three common seated positions:

1 comfortable pose

Tuck each foot under its opposite leg and rest your hands on your knees. In this and in all seated positions, you may use a firm pillow or folded blanket beneath your hips for support. If your back rounds, use a thicker pillow or blanket.

2 accomplished pose

Fold your legs to bring your heels towards the centre of your body as shown. Keep your back straight and tall, your shoulders relaxed and low, and your chin parallel to the floor. Relax your face and jaw and rest your hands comfortably.

3 half lotus pose

Take care doing this challenging pose. Lift one foot and place it on its opposite thigh, sole up, close to your hip. Tuck the other foot under its opposite thigh.

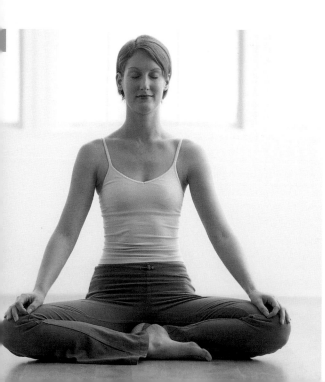

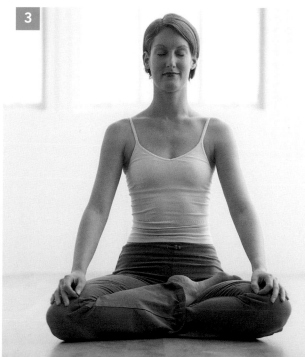

sun salutation Yoga practice often starts with this classic *vinyasa*,

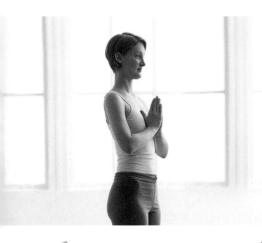 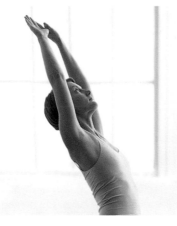 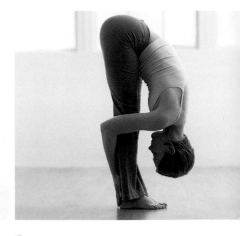

1 praying mountain

Stand tall with your hands in prayer position, feet together, weight evenly on both feet. With your shoulders low and loose, elongate your spine. Exhale.

2 backward bend

Extend your arms forwards, then inhale, lift up your arms by your ears and gently arch your upper back backwards. Don't drop your head; keep your lower back long.

3 forward bend

Exhale and fold forwards from your hips. To intensify the stretch, hold behind your legs and pull your chest towards them. To ease it, bend your knees; let your head and arms hang.

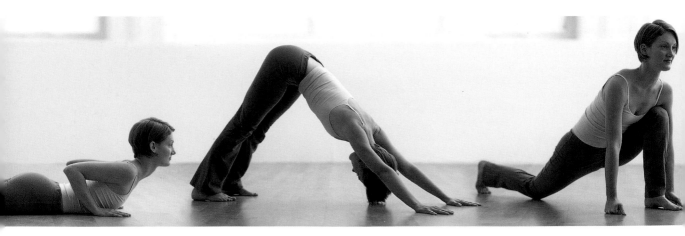

7 cobra

Holding your breath, press into your palms and slide your chest forwards, until you lie flat. With no hand pressure, arch your head, neck and chest.

8 downward dog

Keeping your hands and feet in place, press down on your palms, exhaling as you lift your hips. Press your chest towards your feet and heels towards the floor.

9 lunge

Inhale and swing your left foot between your hands; the left heel is directly under the left knee. Lower your right knee to the floor, and rest your palms or fists on the floor.

or series of flowing poses, which thoroughly engages the body in a balanced way.

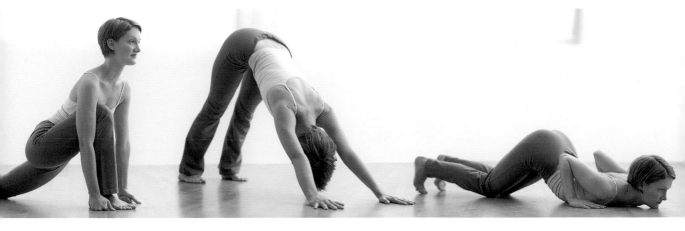

4 lunge

Place palms or fists beside your feet. Inhale and step your left leg back, lowering your left knee to the floor; keep your right knee directly over your right heel.

5 downward dog

Exhaling, step your right foot beside your left. Straighten your knees, sink your heels down and lift your hips. Press into your palms, elongating your back.

6 spider

Inhale and gently lower your knees to the floor. With your hips lifted, place your chest and chin on the floor. Keep your shoulders back and arms close beside your ribs.

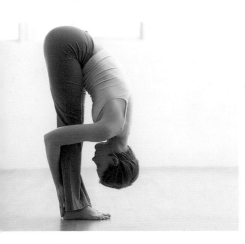

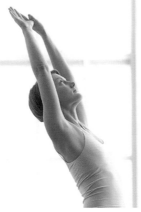

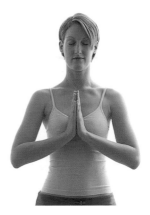

10 forward bend

Exhale as you bring your right foot forwards beside your left and straighten your knees. To ease the stretch, bend your knees and let your head and arms hang.

11 backward bend

Extend your arms, flatten your back and inhale as you rise to standing (bend your knees if you need to protect your back). Arch just your upper back backwards.

12 praying mountain

Exhale as you return to the starting pose. In the next set, step your right leg back in step 4 and forward in step 9. Try 2–3 Sun Salutations as a warm-up or 5–10 as a daily practice.

radiance

When we first wake, we have a natural instinct to stretch, to revive and invigorate our bodies. Honour that inclination by making time for yoga. Morning practice eases the stiffness that settles into your muscles as you sleep and validates your commitment to your wellbeing. It's the perfect way to prepare both mind and body for a radiant and vibrant day.

key benefits

- ▶ Affirms mental and physical wellbeing
- ▶ Wakes up stiff, sleepy muscles
- ▶ Sets you up for a bright day

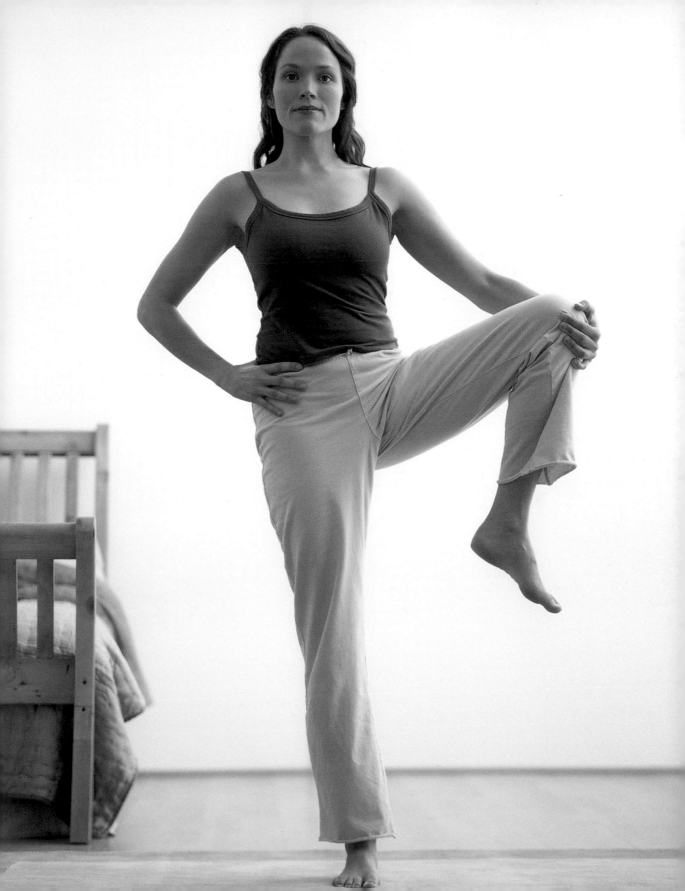

awaken and energise

Start your day off well with some standing yoga poses that will loosen up sleep-tightened muscles and get you charged up for the day ahead.

Wake Up and Smell the Mint Tea
Excessive consumption of caffeinated drinks can put stress on your adrenal glands and nervous system, causing extra wear and tear on your body and setting your mind racing. Instead of getting a caffeine jolt in the morning, encourage alertness with aromatic alternatives. Peppermint gently stimulates your body while calming the mind. Sweet orange lifts your mood, increasing radiance and joy. To feel calm as well as energised, try a warm cup of mint or orange tea, or use body products containing peppermint or sweet orange essential oil.

1 crescent moon

Standing with your feet together, interlace your fingers, pointing your index fingers upwards. Lift your arms overhead and inhale, elongating your spine. Exhale, moving your hips to your left and your hands to the right. Feel the arch from your feet to your fingertips. Do not let your chest roll forwards. Breathe into your upraised side. Hold for four breaths, then inhale and release. Repeat on the other side.

2 standing camel

Place your hands on your hips and roll your shoulders back, moving your shoulder blades towards each other. Tighten your buttocks and move your hips forwards, keeping your lower back flat. Inhaling, lift your chest and arch your upper back. Do not allow your head to drop. Hold for several breaths, eventually releasing on an inhalation.

3 hip hug

Shift your weight to your right foot, tightening the front of your right thigh. Inhale, then bring your left knee towards your chest as you exhale. Hold for a few breaths, coaxing your leg up and in. Then wrap your left hand around your left knee, place your right hand on your right hip and open your left leg to the side (see page 19 ◄). Hold for a few breaths. Release and repeat with the other leg.

4 wide warrior

Stand with your feet about 90 to 120 cm apart. Point your left (front) foot forwards and your right (back) foot slightly right, keeping your heels in line with each other. Hold your arms out to your sides and parallel to the floor, palms down, and look left as you inhale. Keeping your spine vertical, exhale and bend your left knee, bringing it over your heel. Try to lower your left thigh until it is parallel with the floor; you may need to adjust the width of your stance. Hold for 4–10 breaths. Release and repeat the pose on the other side.

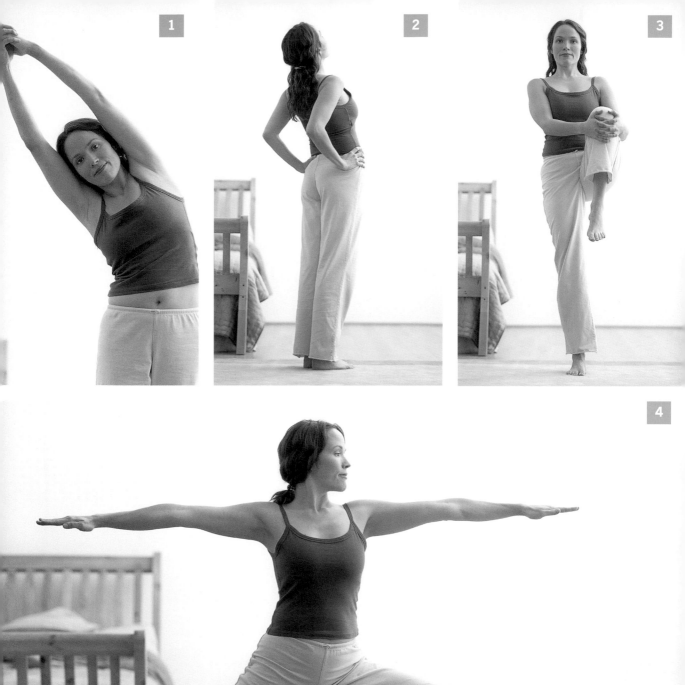

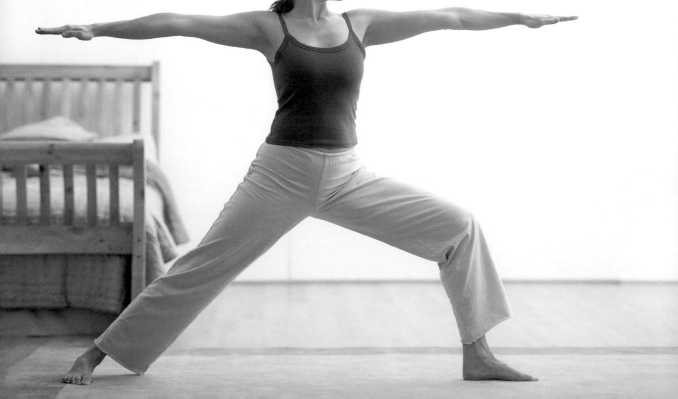

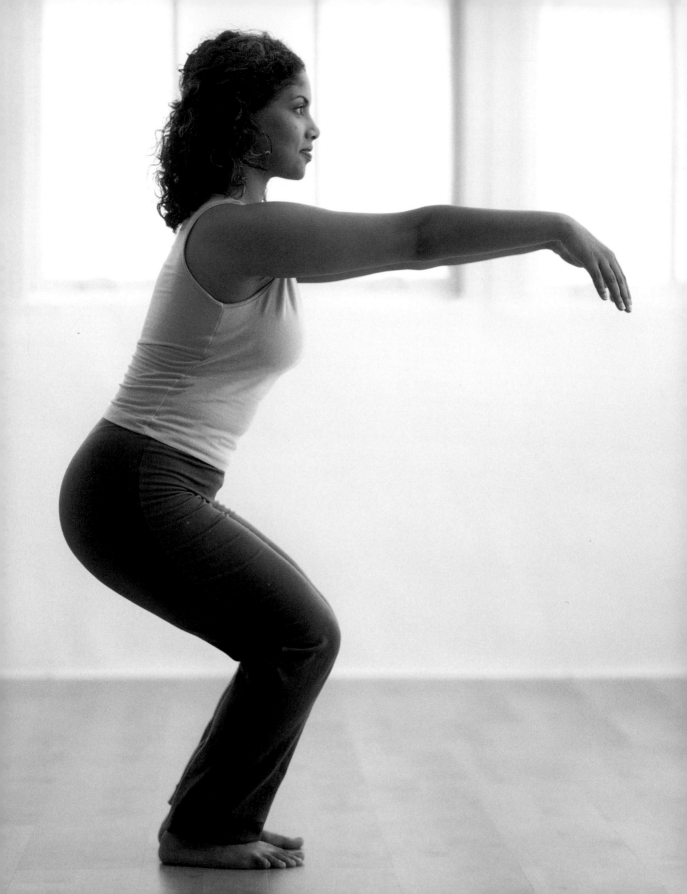

vigour

Many of us work to enhance our strength using machines or weights. But building strength with yoga is unique, because all you need is your body, willpower, and some floor and wall space. Performing these poses is intense, rewarding and graceful work. It will leave you feeling invigorated, engaged and alive.

key benefits

- ▶ Increases strength
- ▶ Tones legs, abdomen and upper body
- ▶ Boosts energy levels

vigour

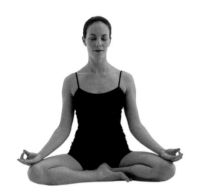

Victory Breath
Ujjayi, also called the Victory Breath, helps to stabilise body and mind by adding control to the flow of your breath. The practice consists of breathing slowly and deeply while partially closing the top of your throat, as you would if exhaling to fog a mirror. You will hear a light hissing sound as you breathe. The Victory Breath is especially useful during challenging poses; feel the discipline of your breath calming and strengthening your efforts.

inner strength

These classic poses are core moves for strength building. As you practise these poses, look for your edge: the point of maximum effort without strain.

1 tall warrior

With your feet 90 to 120 cm apart, point your right (front) foot forwards and your left (back) foot slightly left. Keep your heels in line with each other and square your hips towards your right foot. Bring your arms overhead and inhale. As you exhale, bend your right leg until your knee is over your heel. Tighten the front of your left thigh. Hold for 4–10 breaths. Release. Repeat on the other side.

2 supported chair

Standing against a wall with your feet hip-distance apart, inhale, lifting your arms parallel to the floor and keeping your wrists relaxed. Exhaling, slide your back down the wall as you step your feet forwards. Keep your hips higher than your knees and your knees directly above your heels. Hold for about 30 seconds and release.

3 supported forward boat

Sitting on the floor with your knees bent, place your hands on the back of your thighs near your knees. Lift your lower back inwards and upwards. Keeping your back muscles engaged, exhale and lean backwards, letting your legs lift to challenge your abdominal muscles. Hold for up to 30 seconds, with your calves parallel to the floor. Release, lowering your legs and back to the floor, and relax.

4 dolphin

Kneel and grasp each upper arm with the opposite hand, placing your elbows on the floor. Keeping your elbows in place, release your hands and interlace your fingers in front of you. Press down with your arms and lift your hips. Keep your back straight, inhale and move your chin out past your hands. Exhale and bring your head inside your arms. Continue for several repetitions. (See pages 26–27 ▶ for more challenging versions of Chair, Boat and Dolphin.)

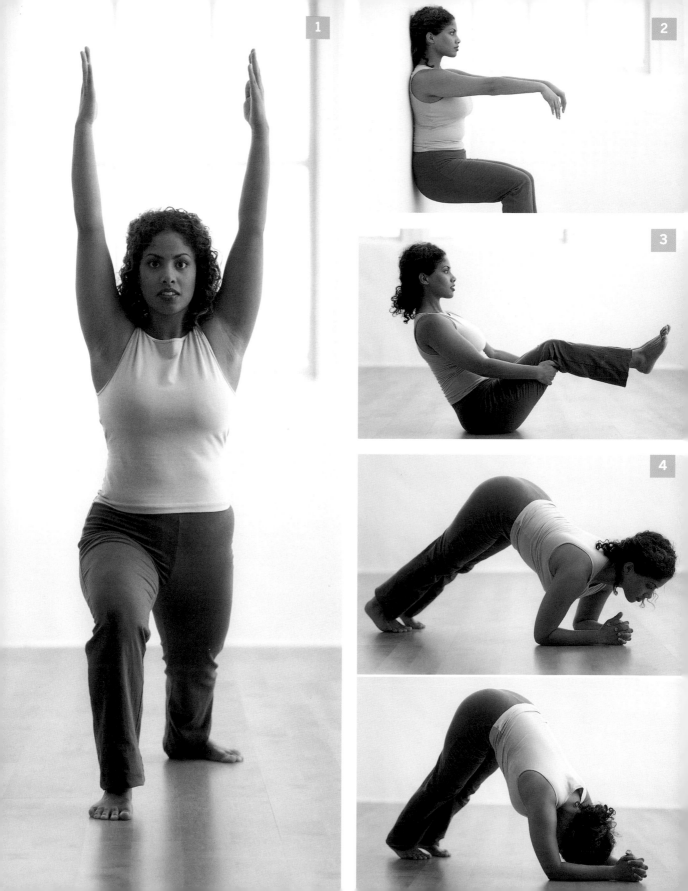

watch yourself

Self-awareness is one benefit of practising yoga. Learn to observe your body, watching it as it changes, and vary your practice according to your body's needs.

These variations are more intense versions of the poses in the main sequence on the preceding pages. Take care not to push yourself beyond your limits; choose a version of an asana based on the wisdom of your body rather than on the desires of your ego to achieve more.

Practise *satya* (truthfulness) and *santosha* (contentment) in regard to your physical abilities. Be patient. Working at, but not striving beyond, the edge of your ability is the ideal way to build strength.

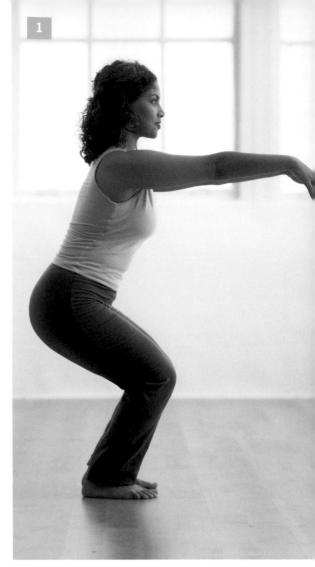

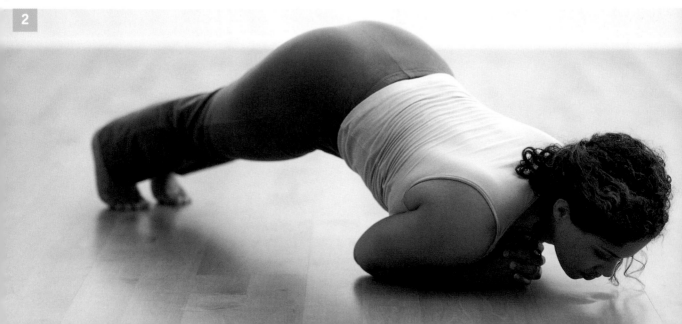

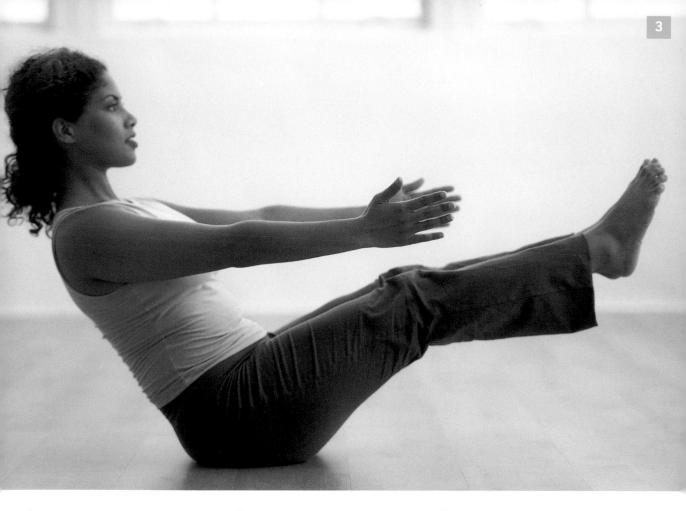

3

1 freestanding chair

With your feet hip-distance apart, inhale and lift your arms parallel to the floor, wrists relaxed. Exhale, bend your knees and lower your hips, keeping them higher than your knees. Don't overarch your lower back; sink down and back into your hips. Hold for 4–10 breaths. If this is comfortable, try holding this pose on your tiptoes, then on your tiptoes with your knees touching. Practise all three variations to fully work your quadriceps (front thigh muscles).

2 deep dolphin

To intensify the Dolphin pose (see page 24 ◄), try to touch your chin to the floor when you move your head past your hands. As you move your head back inside your arms, try to touch your forehead to the floor. Keep your shoulders wide and press your elbows down firmly to prevent slipping. As this pose grows easier, you may try increasing the number of repetitions. Rest in the Child pose (see page 87 ►) afterwards.

3 full forward boat

Begin in Supported Forward Boat (see page 24 ◄), then release your hands. If your back and legs remain steady, hold the pose with your arms parallel to the floor, thumbs up. Hold for 4–10 breaths. To further intensify, extend and straighten your legs. If you feel strain at any point, go back to an easier version, or release and rest.

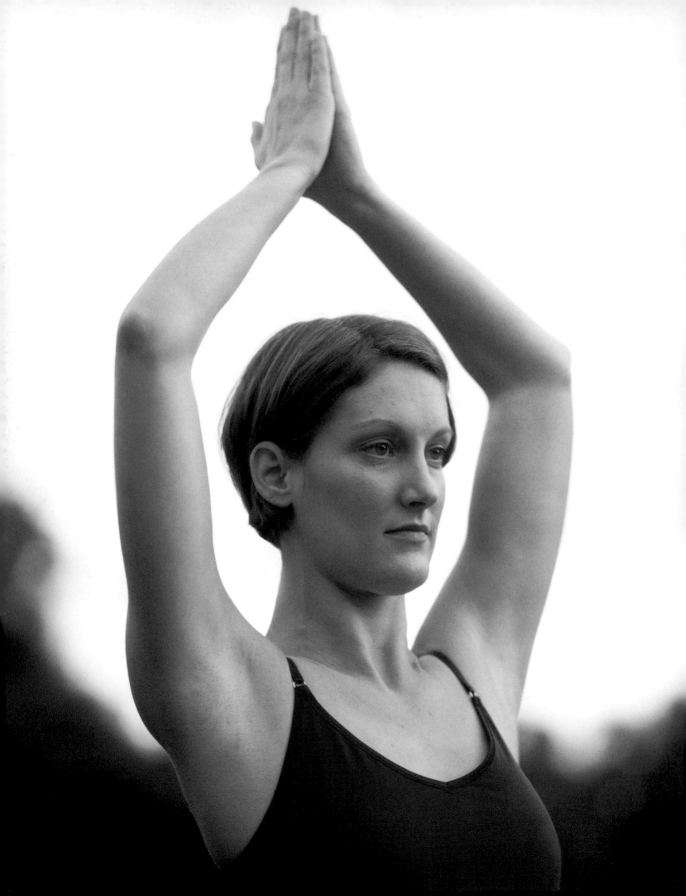

grace

Grace is a process, a dynamic interaction between body and mind. Yoga poses that focus on balance let you play with movement and stillness, helping to build physical strength and mental acuity and increasing the connection between thought and action. Finding your equilibrium will bring increased confidence and poise.

key benefits

▶ Tightens the mind–body connection

▶ Improves balance and coordination

▶ Enhances physical and mental poise

grace

strive for balance

Practising these poses regularly will help you feel centred and well balanced. They can also foster powerful feelings of calmness and control.

Find Your Centre

- When balancing, fix your gaze on a point at or below eye level in front of you. Visualise a triangle of stability between that point of focus, your eyes and your centre of gravity (just below your navel).
- Thinking of your foot as a single point of balance can cause you to overwork. Imagine that your foot is a suspension bridge. Lift and support its arch with weight distributed between your heel, the base of your big toe and the base of your little toe. Using these three points of support helps you achieve a solid base.

1 mountain

A stable Mountain pose is the starting point for all standing poses. Stand with your feet together and your arms relaxed at your sides; tighten your quadriceps (at the front of your thighs) to stabilise your knees. Hold for several breaths, feeling the steadiness and calm of a mountain. Close your eyes to see how that affects your balance.

2 tree

Shift your weight to your left leg, then place your right foot on the inside of your left leg as high as you comfortably can (avoid putting it directly on the inside of your knee). Bring your palms together in front of your heart. Rotate your bent leg back so it's in the same plane as your chest. Hold for ten breaths and release. Then repeat this pose on the other leg. (See page 32 ► for an easier variation.)

3 king dancer

Shift your weight to your right leg, then lift your left foot behind you and grasp it with your left hand. Lift your right arm overhead, palm forwards, and inhale, arching your back gently. Press your left foot backwards into your hand and breathe evenly. Keep your right arm beside your right ear and pivot forwards from the top of your right leg. Hold for ten breaths, release and repeat on the other side. (If it's hard to hold this pose, try the variations on page 33 ►).

4 warrior

Lift your arms overhead as you inhale, then exhale and step forwards with your right leg and pivot forwards, lifting your left leg and lowering your chest. Keep your body in a straight line from heel to fingertips; your chest and leg may be parallel to the floor, nearly upright, or anywhere in between – find what's comfortable for you. If you feel shaky, bend your standing leg slightly; to ease your back, extend your arms out to your sides instead of overhead. Hold for several breaths, releasing on an inhalation. Repeat on the other leg.

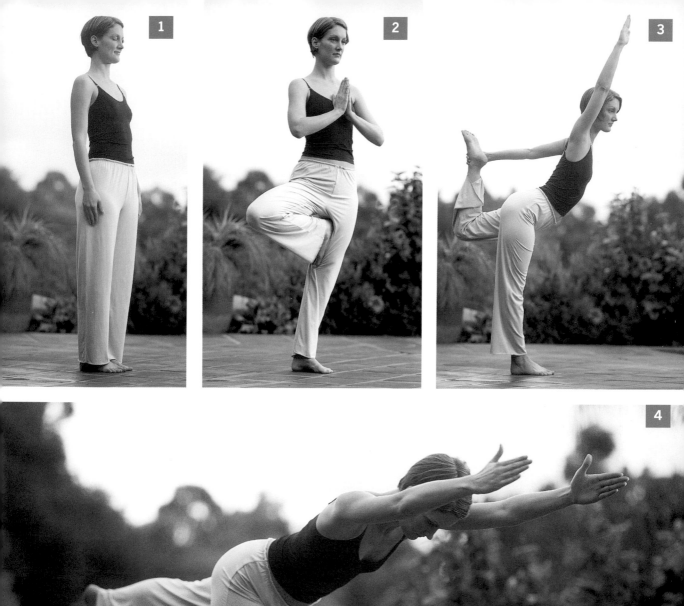
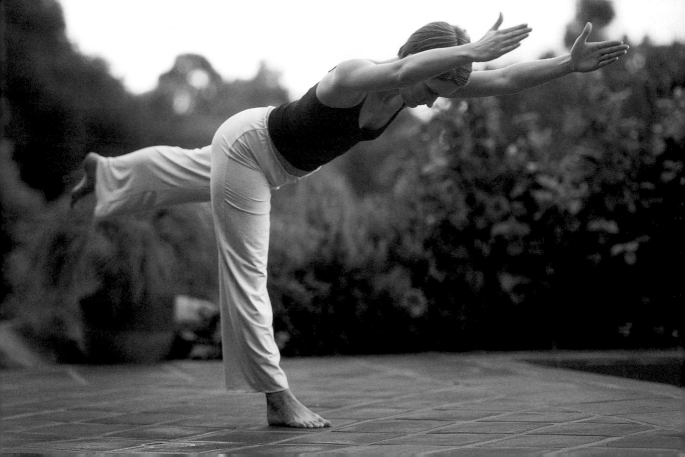

get steady

When practising standing and balancing poses, you strive to feel the solidity of the Mountain pose (page 30 ◄). But sometimes you may need help feeling steady. Practising near or against a wall offers a sense of safety as you find your equilibrium. Be sure to work both sides.

Remember that as you practise, you don't need to be perfectly steady to increase your strength and harmony. In yoga, the quality of your effort is what is important – and it is also what brings the results that matter. Each step you take towards steadiness adds to your self-knowledge and increases your skill.

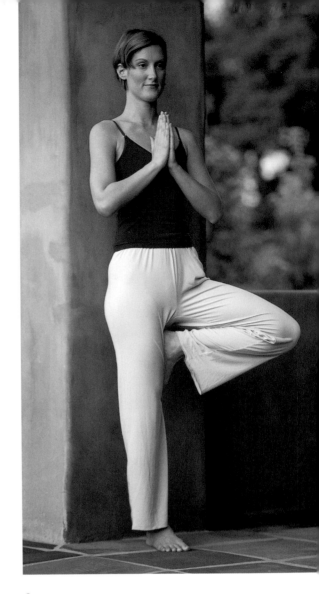

1 tree at the wall

Standing a few centimetres from a wall or another steady surface, lean against it and come into the Tree pose (page 30 ◄). Inhale. As you exhale, slowly shift forwards until you are freestanding and breathe evenly, holding the pose. When this becomes easy, practise standing slightly further away from the wall, using your awareness of it to provide a sense of support. Gradually move further away from the wall until unsupported practice comes naturally.

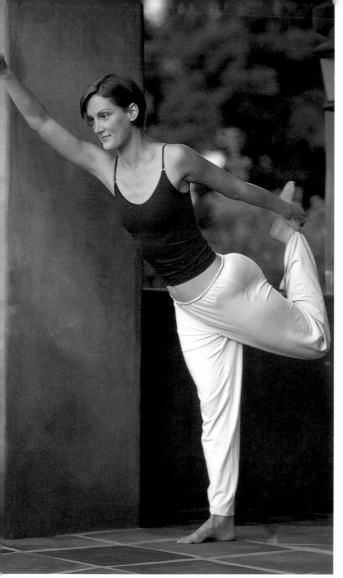

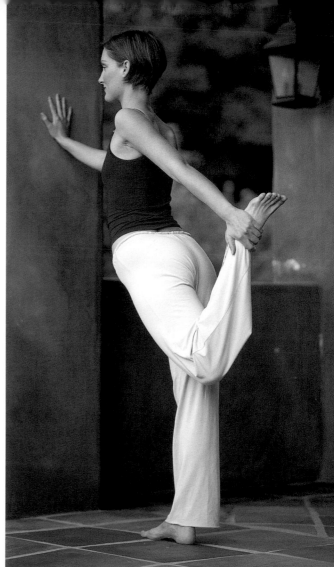

2 dancer along the wall

You can also try the King Dancer pose (page 30 ◄) alongside and close to, but not touching, a wall. Simply hold the pose with the wall at your side. Balance is a mind–body skill, so this mental support is sometimes all you need to give you the confidence that will help you stabilise your body.

3 dancer at the wall

If you'd like to stretch your quadriceps for longer than you can balance, place your free hand on the wall for support as you practise the King Dancer pose (page 30 ◄). Begin with your supporting arm straight, then bend it as you pivot forwards. If you're feeling steady, take your hand from the wall and lift it overhead to practise this pose without support.

release

Releasing tension in your hip joints helps give you a greater range of movement, soothes your lower back and brings increased comfort to your movements. It also can be rewarding emotionally. Intense experiences can be stored in the body as tension, and loosening up that tightness can lighten your mind in surprising ways.

key benefits

▶ Relieves tension in hips and back

▶ Lightens your mood

▶ Increases range of movement

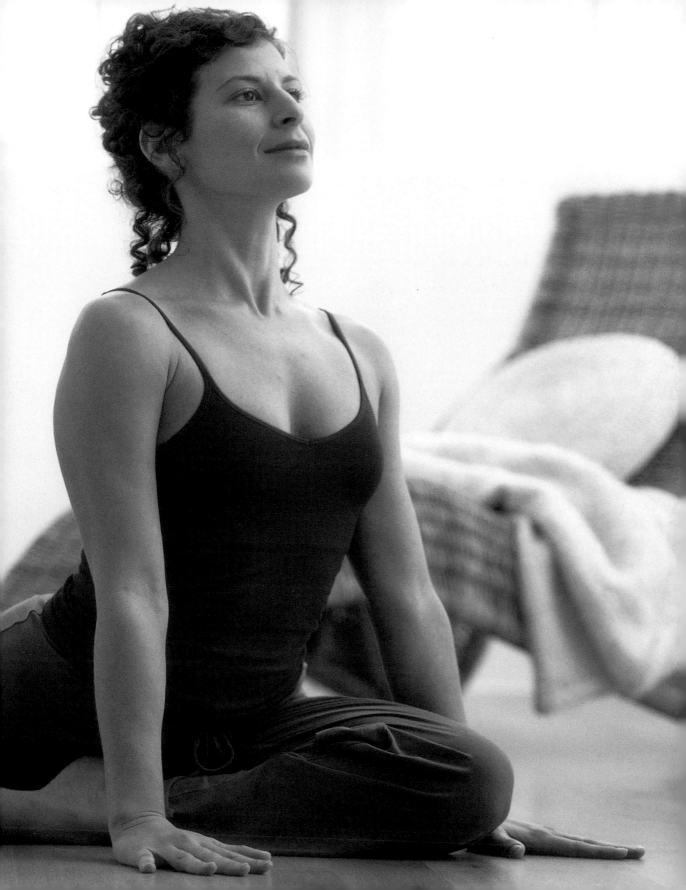

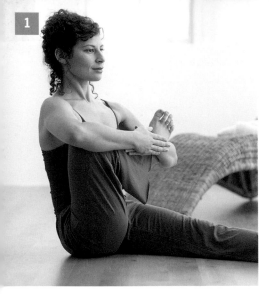

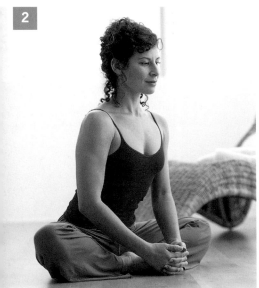

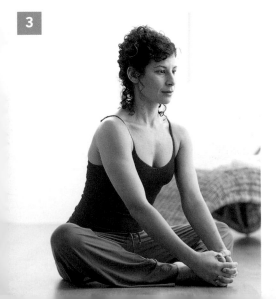

expand your range

Reap the physical and emotional benefits of more flexible hips. As you go through these poses, pay attention to your body and don't push beyond your comfort level.

1 rock the baby

Sit with both legs extended in front of you, then bend your right knee and lift that leg towards your chest. Sitting as straight as you can, hug your leg inwards and gently rock it side to side, as you would rock a baby, to increase flexibility in your hip. Ideally your elbows will wrap around your knee and foot, but use any grasp that is comfortable. Practise for 4–8 breaths, release and repeat with the other leg.

2 cobbler

Bring the soles of your feet together and grasp your feet or ankles. Sit straight and gently press your knees towards the floor. To intensify, inhale and elongate your spine, then exhale, leaning forwards from your hips. Keep your head in line with your spine and continue to elongate with each inhalation, sinking slightly deeper towards the floor with each exhalation. Hold for 30 seconds, then release.

3 forward cobbler

To stretch the back of your hips, slide your feet forwards about 30 cm and repeat the forward bend; your arms will bend less in this version. (If your arms can touch your legs in either version of Cobbler, use your elbows or forearms to gently press against your calves and increase the stretch.) Focus your mind on the point where the stretch is most intense and visualise it softening. Hold for 30 seconds.

4 thread the needle

Lie on your back with your left leg bent, knee pointed upwards. Place your right ankle on your left thigh just below your knee, taking care to keep your right foot flexed. Grasp the back of your left thigh with both hands and pull it gently towards your chest. To intensify the stretch, try pressing your right leg away with your right elbow as you continue to pull your left leg towards you. Hold for 4–8 breaths. Release and repeat the pose with the other leg.

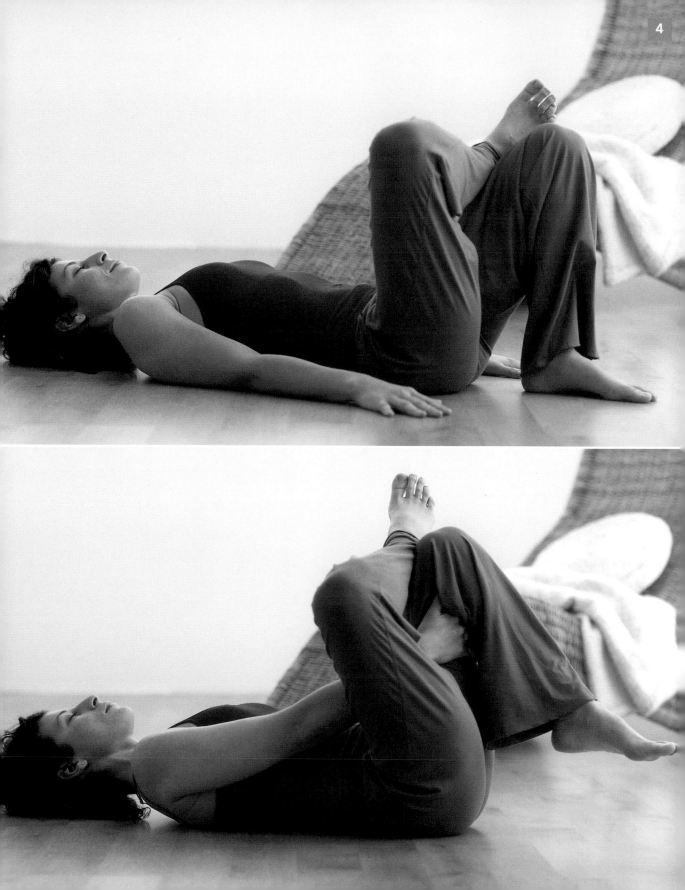

pigeon practice

These variations of the Pigeon pose provide more challenging opportunities to work on releasing your hips.

Your hips work in harmony with your knees, which may try to compensate for restrictions in the range of motion of your hip joints. When challenging your hip joints, take care that you are not creating strain in your knees. Release any pose at the first sign of strain.

Remember that yoga practice does not end when you leave your mat; observe how your body is affected by your practice immediately afterwards and, as you practise regularly, over time.

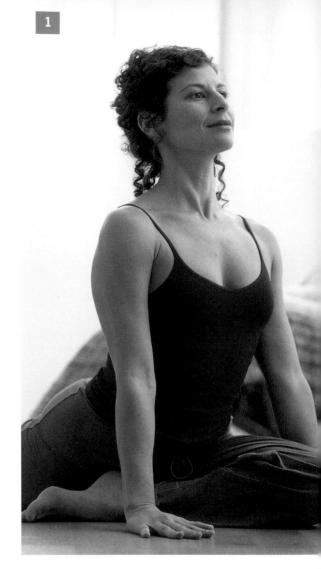

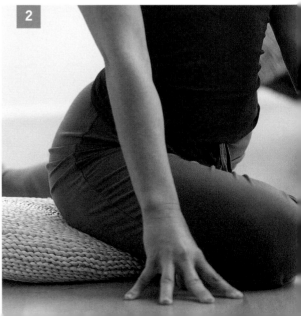

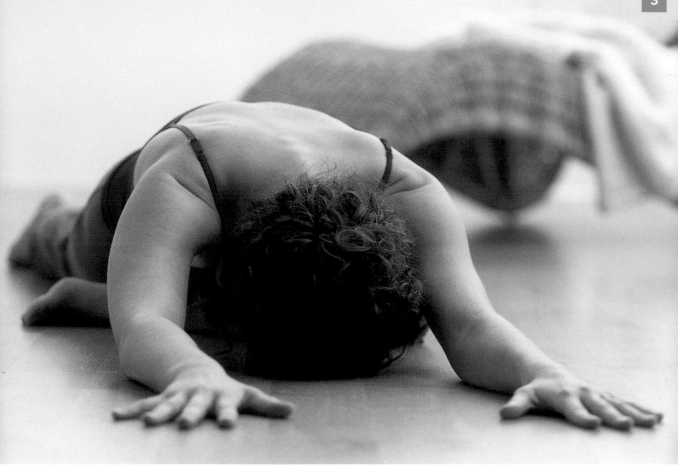

1 pigeon

Starting on all fours, bring your left knee forwards so it is between your hands, with your foot to the right so that your leg forms an inverted V. Extend your right leg back and allow your hips to sink, keeping them level with the floor; do not roll onto your left thigh. Elongate your spine, lift your chest, and keep your shoulders loose and low. Hold the pose for 4–6 breaths. To release, push down with your palms, lift your hips and slide your left leg back. Repeat the pose on the other side.

2 supported pigeon

If you find it difficult to keep your hips level in either the Pigeon or the Low Pigeon pose, place a firm pillow or a folded blanket under the hip of the bent-leg side. The further your hips are from the floor, the thicker the pillow or blanket needs to be. With regular practice, you will gradually need less support.

3 low pigeon

From the Pigeon pose (pose 1), relax down over your bent leg. Lower your weight onto your forearms, placing them on the floor shoulder-width apart. If this is comfortable, release more weight onto your bent leg by extending your arms completely and letting your head rest on (or hang towards) the floor. Notice the places where your body is resisting and try to surrender. Hold the pose for 4–6 breaths. Repeat Low Pigeon on the other side.

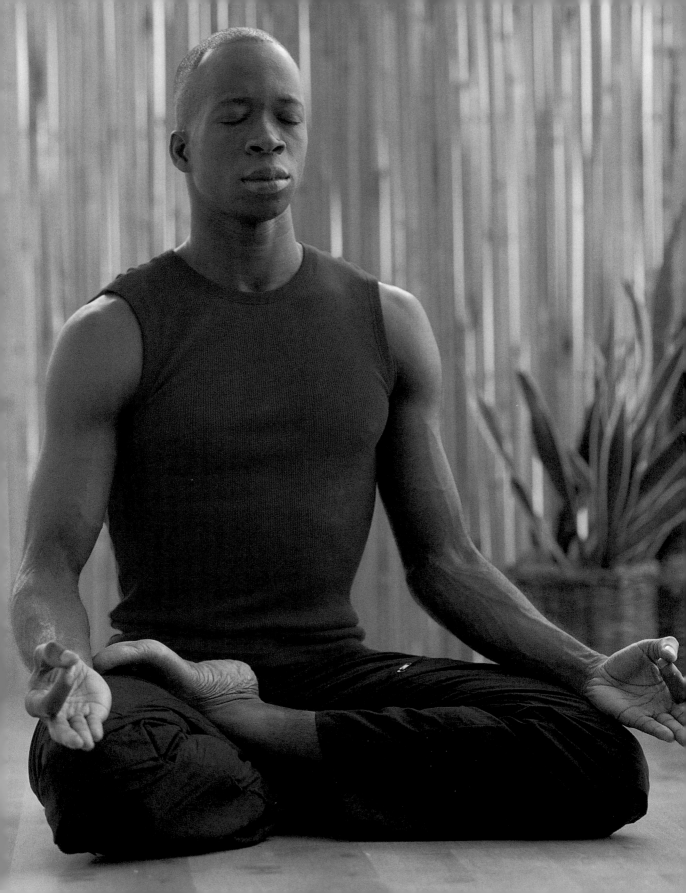

clarity

When your mind is calm, it functions more effectively and life is more enjoyable. But daily stresses can create tension in your upper body, clouding your thoughts and causing discomfort and even headaches. A few gentle movements can help alleviate the tightness in your head, neck and shoulders – leaving you feeling both physically relaxed and mentally clear.

key benefits

▶ Eases tension in head, neck and shoulders

▶ Alleviates headaches

▶ Improves concentration and mental sharpness

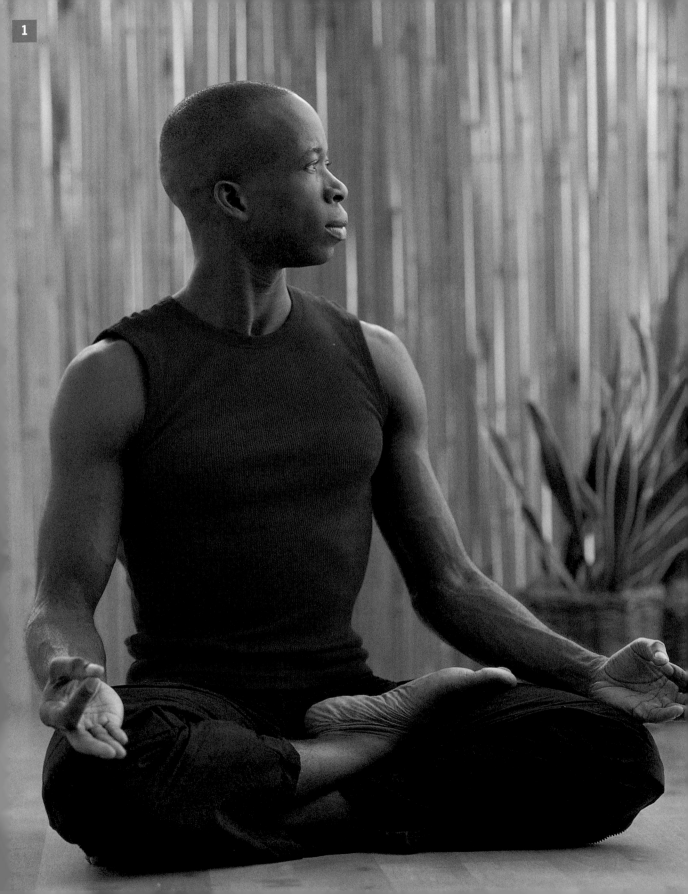

get a head start

Find a quiet corner to perform these seated yoga
postures, which will help release upper-body tension,
boost concentration and sharpen clarity of thought.

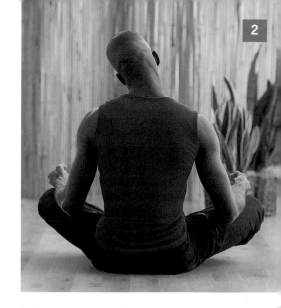

1 gazing rotation

From a seated position (see page 15 ◄), inhale and lengthen your
spine. Keeping your chin level, exhale as you turn to look over
your left shoulder. Continue to rotate your head as you feel your
shoulders and neck relax. Focus your mind on becoming completely
present in your body and try to set thoughts aside. Hold for four
breaths, then inhale as you return to centre. Repeat on the other side.

2 wilting blossom

Inhaling, drop your shoulders as you lift the crown of your head
towards the ceiling. Exhaling, lower your left ear towards your left
shoulder. Hold for four breaths, gently increasing the distance
between the top of your head and your right shoulder. Release on
an inhalation, then repeat, lowering your head to the right.

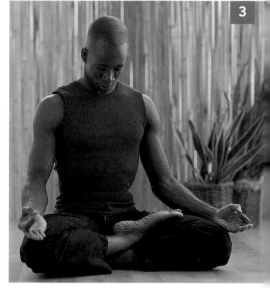

3 neck rolls

Exhale as you lower your chin to your chest, then inhale and roll
your right ear towards your right shoulder. Exhale and roll your head
down to centre, then inhale and roll your left ear towards your left
shoulder. Continue gently rolling from shoulder to shoulder at the
pace of your breath. Visualise weariness or everyday stress leaving
your body with each exhalation and peace and vitality entering
with each inhalation. Continue rolling for six breaths; then, on an
inhalation, raise your head up and relax.

4 shoulder rolls

On an inhalation, lift your shoulders towards your ears and then roll
them back and downwards on an exhalation. Inhale forwards and up
and exhale back and down, making the deepest circles you can for
four breaths; then reverse direction. Keep your shoulders broad as
you roll, taking care that you do not lean forwards.

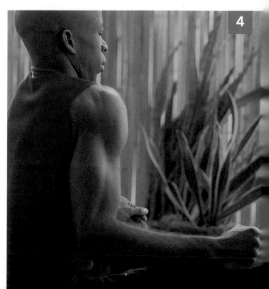

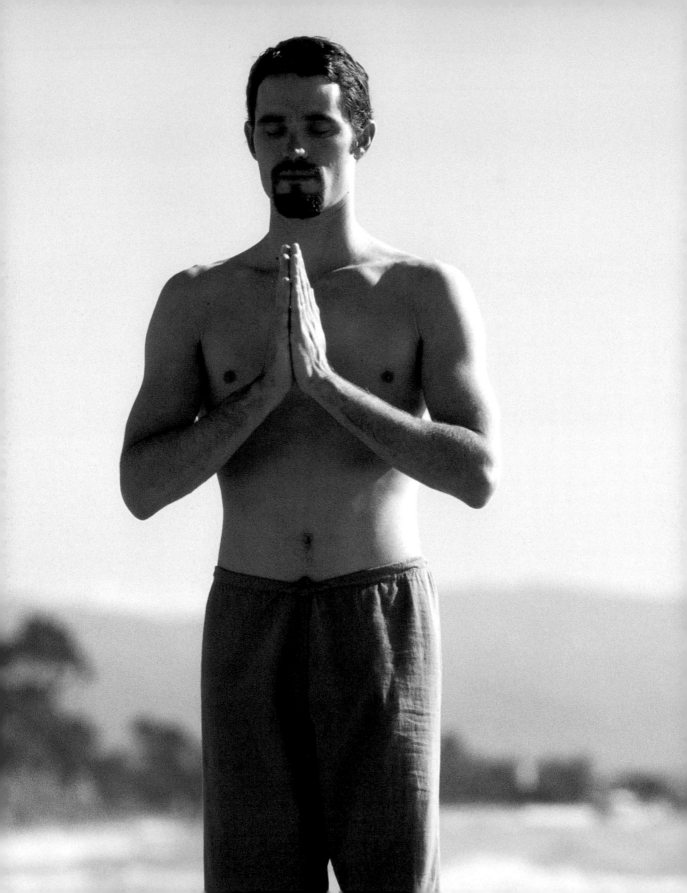

serenity

According to yogic teaching, serenity is our natural state of being, always present within each of us. Practising yoga can help you free yourself from the clutter of everyday stress and worry, allowing your inner calm to shine through. Cultivate *sat-chit-ananda*, the bliss that arises simply from the awareness of being.

key benefits

▶ Helps you become more present in the moment

▶ Calms your mind

▶ Helps you think more clearly

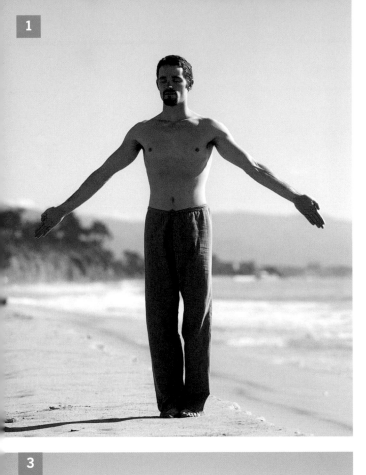

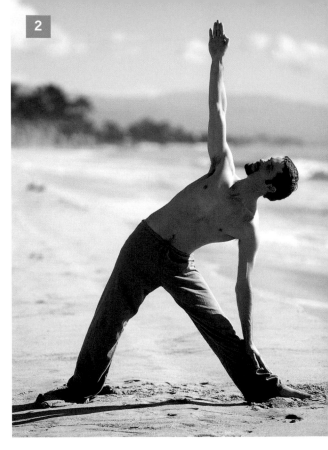

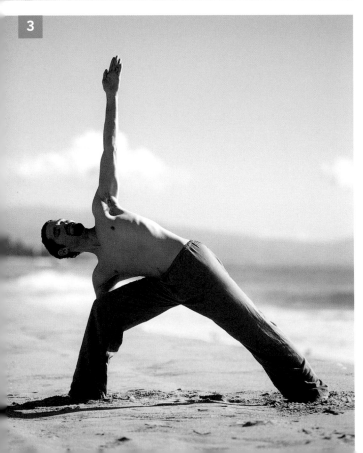

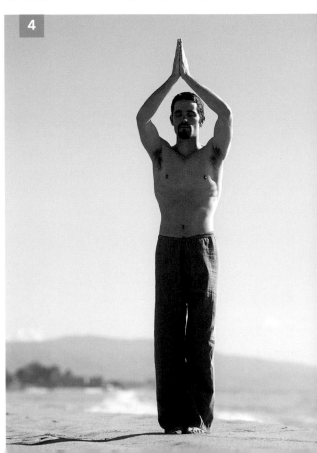

let your spirit soar

Whether you do them in your bedroom or on the beach, these poses will help you quiet everyday worries and bolster a sense of serenity and peace.

1 funnel

Stand with your feet together and your palms together in a prayer position at your heart (see photo at right). Inhaling, lower your hands until they part, then exhale and sweep them out to your sides and upwards. Join them together overhead, then inhale, draw them back down and repeat. Imagine funnelling a current of light into your body as you repeat these circles for several breaths.

2 triangle

Step about a leg's length apart. Turn your right foot slightly left and your left foot out 90 degrees, keeping your heels in line. With hips facing forwards, lift your arms out to the side, parallel to the ground, palms down. Inhaling, reach left and out. Exhaling, bend sideways to your left. Put your left hand on your leg and your right arm straight up. Look up. Hold for 5–10 breaths. Repeat on the other side.

3 extended wide angle

Turn your right foot out 90 degrees and your left foot slightly right. Exhale and bend your right knee, placing your right palm or fist on the ground behind your foot. (If it's more comfortable, rest your right elbow near the knee of your bent leg instead.) Hold your left arm straight up, palm forwards, and gaze at it or look forwards. Roll your chest upwards and hold for 5–10 breaths. Repeat on the other side.

4 fountain

Stand with your feet together and your palms together in a prayer position at your heart, then inhale and raise your hands overhead, drawing energy upwards. Exhaling, sweep your hands open, wide and down to your sides in a circular motion (the reverse of Funnel). Imagine drawing energy upwards with each inhalation and sending it out in a fountain around your body on each exhalation. Enjoy the lightness of this release of energy as you continue for several breaths.

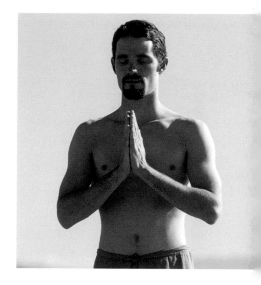

Namaste Mudra

Holding your palms together in prayer position forms an energy seal called *namaste mudra*. The Sanskrit word *namaste*, traditionally spoken at greeting and parting, acknowledges the universal spark within, while *mudra* means "seal".

vitality

Yoga can complement other kinds of exercise, including a gym workout. Start your warm-up with some gentle back and leg stretches to focus your thoughts and harness your determination. Add deep breathing and lunges to help keep you in balance, leaving you both physically and mentally stronger.

key benefits

▶ Makes legs, hips and back supple

▶ Strengthens legs and upper body

▶ Clears your mind before you work out

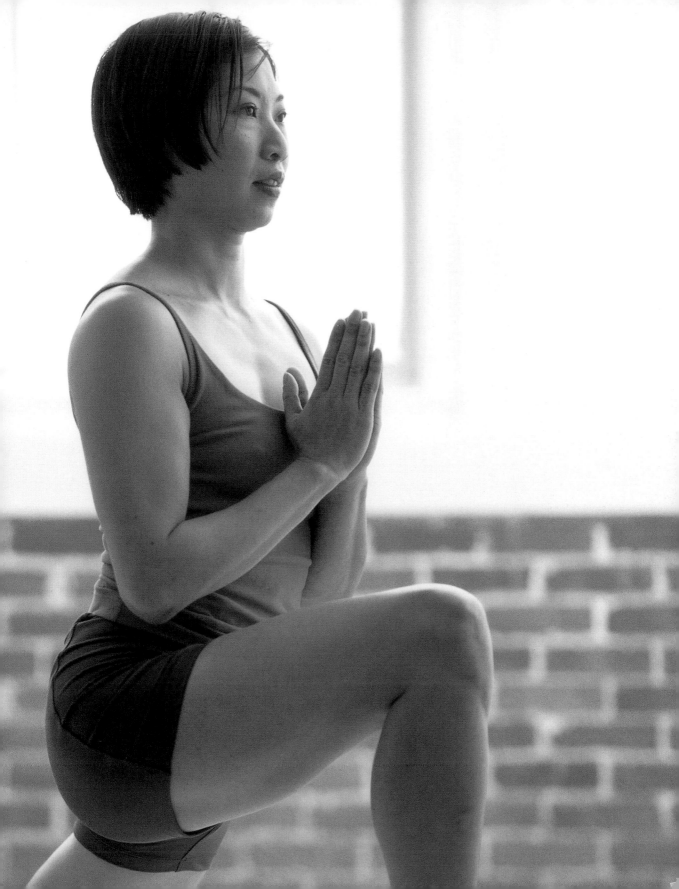

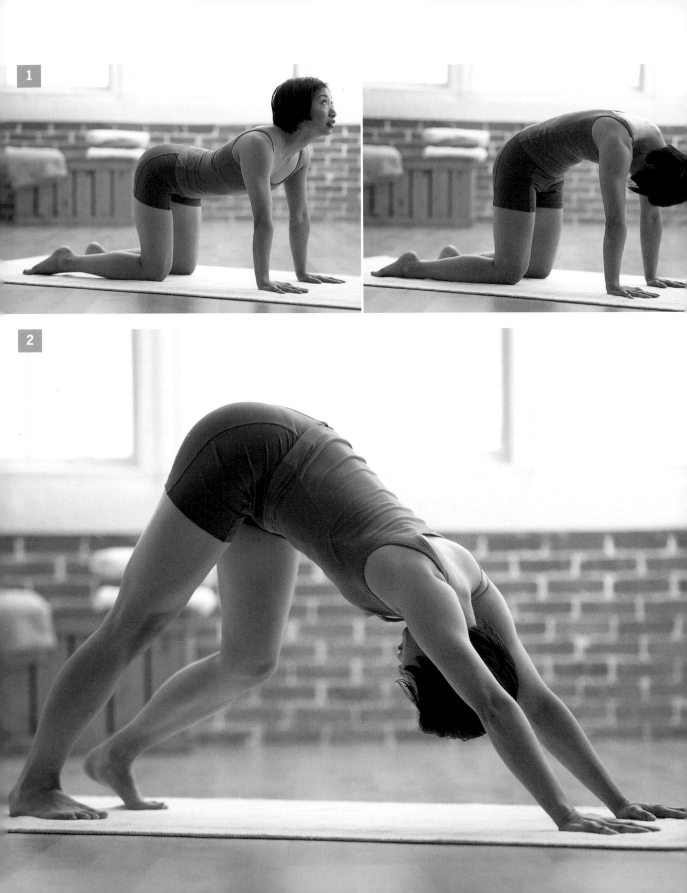

warm up

Find a quiet corner at home or at the gym, unroll
your mat and warm up with some basic moves to
clear your mind and gently loosen tight muscles.

1 cat

To warm up and stretch your back and abdominal muscles, try a
series of Cat stretches. Begin in the Table position: on all fours with
your palms flat directly beneath your shoulders and your knees
directly beneath your hips. (If your wrists are tender, place your
fists down, thumbs forward.) Be careful not to lock your elbows.
Inhale and press your belly down as your chest expands, lifting your
head and tailbone up. Exhale, contracting your diaphragm and
abdomen, while lifting your back up and lowering your head
and tailbone. Repeat for 4–10 breaths.

2 walking downward dog

To warm up your legs as well as your lower back (and strengthen
your upper body at the same time), try a variation of the Downward
Dog pose. As with Cat, start on all fours in Table. Make sure that your
middle fingers are pointing straight forwards. Exhale, lifting your hips
and pressing through your arms out to your fingertips. Lengthen your
back and shoulders as you press your chest towards your feet into the
classic Downward Dog pose (see page 72 ▶). Try to straighten your
knees, let your heels sink towards the floor and allow your head
to hang for a few breaths. For Walking Downward Dog, continue to
press your hands down and your hips upwards while you bend one
knee and push the other heel towards the floor, then reverse sides.
Continue to switch legs using a slow walking motion. Practise for
4–10 breaths. Follow with the Lunge pose (see next page ▶).

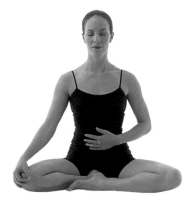

Abdominal Breathing

Whether you're practising a yoga
pose, such as Cat, or jogging on
a treadmill, using your diaphragm to
breathe more deeply can increase
the efficiency of each breath.
Practise abdominal breathing by
placing one hand on your abdomen
just below your ribcage and
expanding your abdomen with each
inhalation, then contracting it with
each exhalation. To help make
abdominal breathing a habit, practise
it for five minutes each day.

go deeper

Once you start to feel warm, try some lunges, which build strength and stretch tight hips. Try these variations as part of the Sun Salutation (see pages 16–17 ◄).

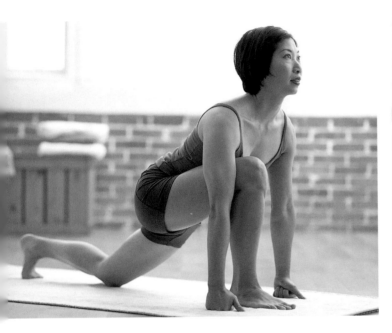

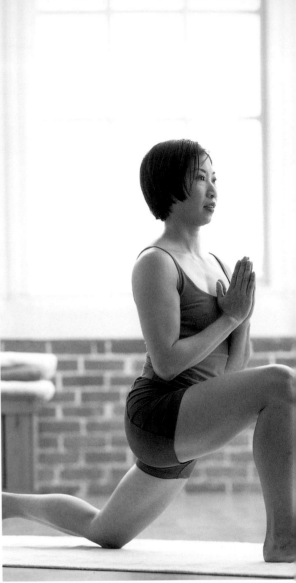

1 lunge

From Downward Dog (see page 51 ◄), exhale and step your right foot between your hands, bringing your left knee to the floor. Make sure your right knee is directly over your heel. (If it's more comfortable, rest your fingertips or fist tops on the floor.) Let your weight sink down into your hips, holding for 4–6 breaths, then step back and push up into Downward Dog. Repeat the pose on your other side.

2 steady monkey

From the preceding Lunge position, lift your chest upright, placing your hands on your front knee for balance. Continue to let your weight sink down into your hips, keeping your shoulders spread wide, back and down. If this is comfortable, try bringing your hands to *namaste mudra* (prayer position, shown) in front of your heart. Hold for 4–10 breaths, then repeat with your other leg in front.

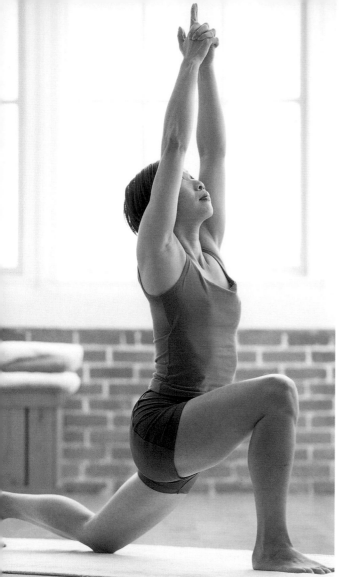

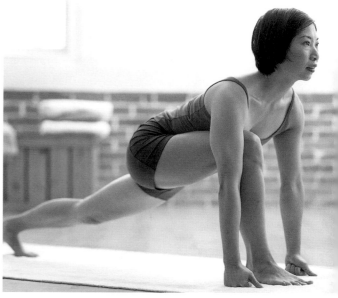

3 tall monkey

From the Steady Monkey pose, lift your arms overhead, interlace your fingers and point your index fingers up while bringing your shoulders back and down. Lengthen and arch your body from your back foot to your fingertips, pressing your hips forward towards your front heel. Gaze up at your fingertips (tilt your head but do not let it drop back too far) and hold for 4–10 breaths. Then repeat the pose with the other leg in front.

4 lifted lunge

From the Lunge position (see pose 1), push out through your back heel and press down with your front leg to lift your back knee off the floor. Keep pressing into your heel, and tighten the front of the thigh of your back leg; feel the back of your knee lifting towards the ceiling. Hold for four breaths, then repeat with your other leg. (If this feels comfortable for you, you can practise all of the Lunge variations with your back leg raised like this to make the poses more challenging.)

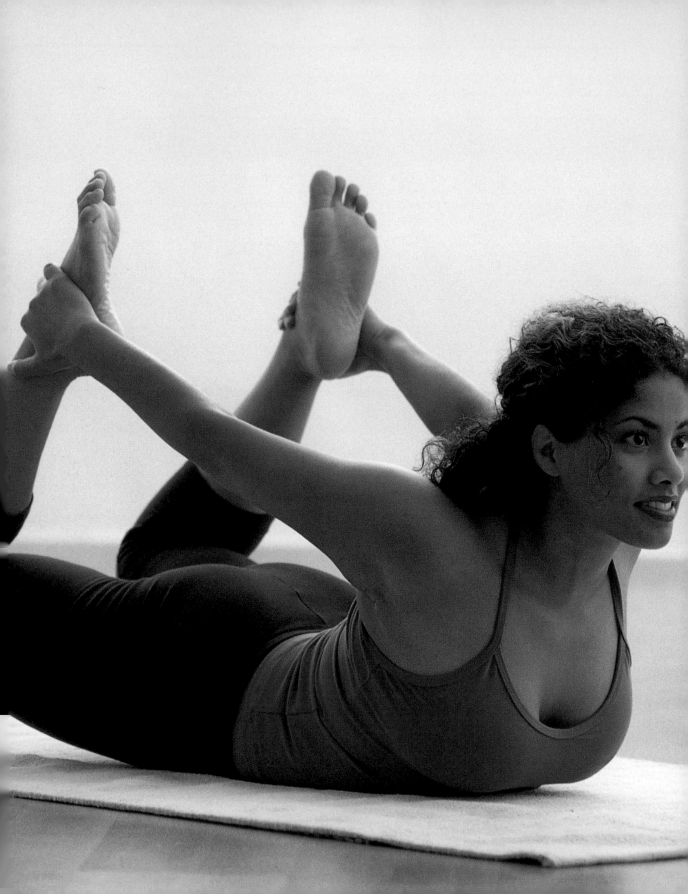

stability

Back muscles are the body's core support, so it's vital to keep them toned and healthy. Backward-bending poses build strength and promote elasticity up and down your spine, while giving abdominal organs a gentle massage. These backbends offer mental benefits, too, because expanding your body can raise your spirits.

key benefits

▶ Helps improve posture

▶ Strengthens vital back muscles

▶ Lifts your mood

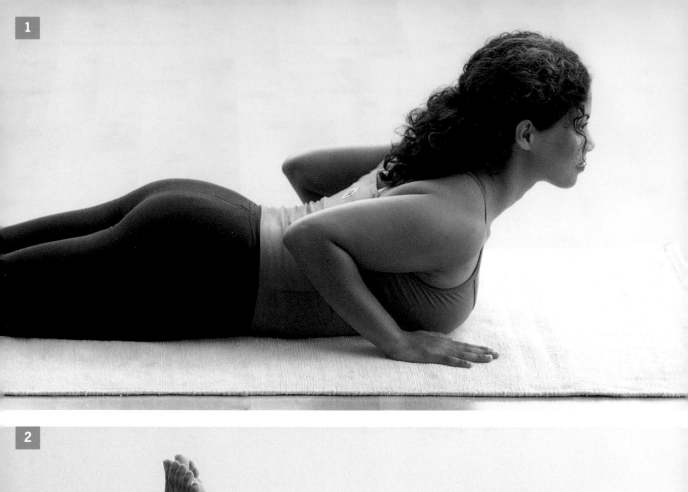

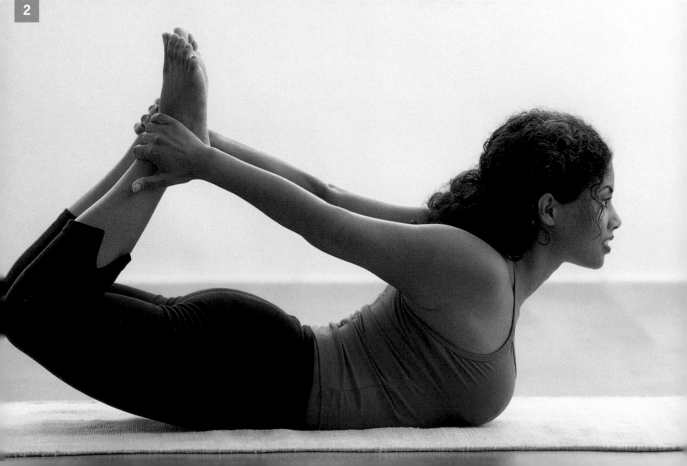

get back to basics

Work out the kinks and increase flexibility up and down your back with these yoga poses that strengthen the back and may even help to improve your posture.

1 cobra

Lie face down with your feet about hip-distance apart, toes pointed back. Place your palms flat on the floor beneath your shoulders, bring your elbows in towards your ribs and rest your forehead on the floor. Inhaling, extend your chin forwards and lift your head, neck and chest as high as you can without putting pressure on your palms. Keep your shoulders low. As you strengthen your upper back, you may feel a physical and emotional release in your chest. Hold the pose for 4–10 breaths before releasing.

2 bow

Bend your knees and reach back to grasp your feet or ankles, whichever is more comfortable. Allow your legs to separate, but keep your heels over your buttocks. Inhaling, raise your head, neck and chest as well as your thighs, pressing your feet into your hands and lifting your heels away from your back. The quality of your effort is more important than how far your body moves. Hold for 4–6 breaths, and exhale as you lower yourself back down to the floor. To release your back, follow with Child and Rabbit (shown at right).

Because abdominal and back muscles work together to provide stability and allow movement at the body's core, keeping a balance between strong back and abdominal muscles is vital. It's best to pair back-strengthening poses, such as Cobra and Bow, with abdominal-strengthening poses, such as Scissors and Blade (see page 61 ▶).

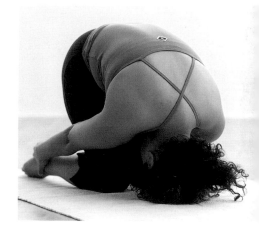

Child and Rabbit
It is important to practise Child and Rabbit as counterposes after backbends such as Cobra and Bow. Bring your buttocks to your heels, forehead to the floor and hands beside your feet, relaxing for three breaths in Child (see page 87 ▶). Then move into Rabbit: grasp your heels, lift your hips and rest the top of your head on the floor. Press out from between your shoulder blades. Hold for 4–6 breaths, then release.

control

Many people strengthen their abdominal muscles for appearance's sake. But strong abdominals are even more important for health. They offer balance for back muscles, aid your digestive system, and may help relieve pain or irregularity in the menstrual cycle. And sustained daily practice – the best approach for gaining strength – builds discipline and self-esteem.

key benefits

▶ Strengthens and tightens abdominal muscles

▶ Balances back muscles for a powerful central core

▶ May help digestion and relieve menstrual pain

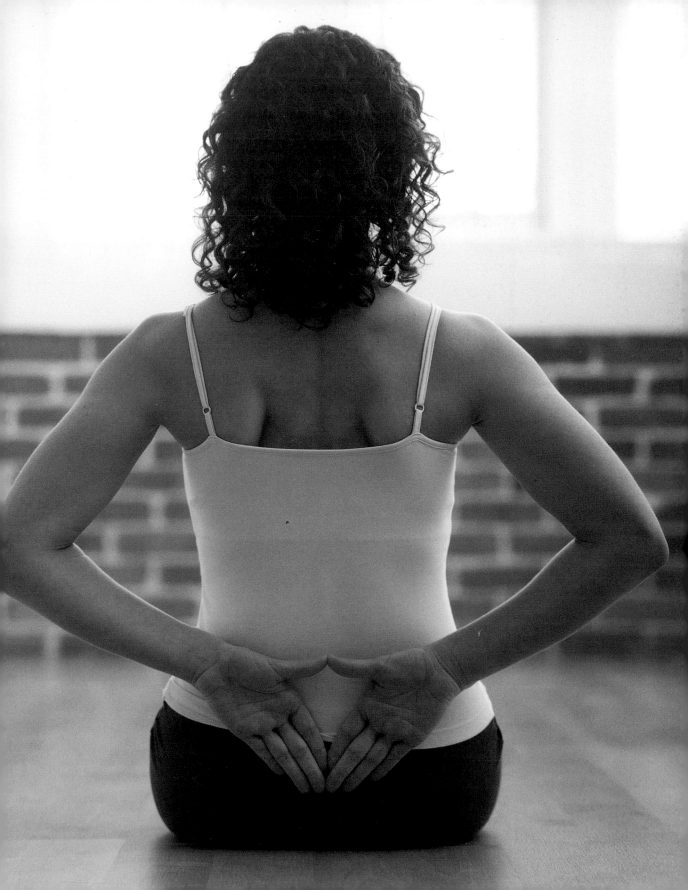

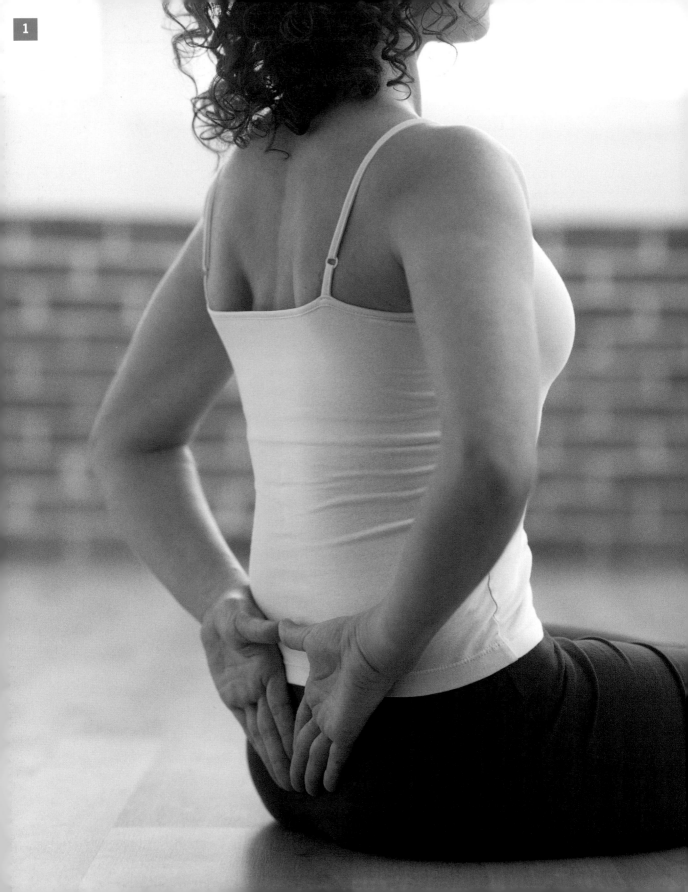

mind your middle

Leg lifts strengthen your abdominal muscles and tone your tummy. Practise at a level that works for you; as you gain more control, step up the intensity.

1 diamond base

This hand position is used to provide support during these poses. Place your hands against your lower back, palms out, with the tips of your thumbs and index fingers touching. (If this makes your shoulders uncomfortable, do these poses with your palms on the floor beside your hips instead.) Throughout these poses, press your lower back down firmly. Stop if your back lifts – an indication of strain.

2 half scissors

Lying on your back, place your left foot on the floor so your bent left knee points upwards. With your right leg straight and your right foot flexed, inhale as you lift your right leg towards the ceiling as high as is comfortable, up to 90 degrees. As you exhale, lower your leg. After lifting and lowering your right leg six times, repeat with your left leg. (You can rest during any of the poses in this sequence by bending your knees and bringing them in against your chest.)

3 scissors

To add challenge to the previous pose, keep your resting leg straight along the floor and alternate legs with each lift. Build intensity gradually; if you feel any strain, go back to Half Scissors. To add even more intensity, hold your resting leg straight up towards the ceiling. After eight lifts with each leg, rest.

4 blade

For the greatest intensity, try lifting and lowering both legs together, inhaling as you lift your legs and exhaling as you lower them, for eight repetitions. When you lower your legs, hold them just above the floor, but not resting on it. As always, stop at any sign of strain. To stretch your abdominals and to strengthen your back muscles for balance before or after doing these poses, practise the Bridge pose (see page 82 ▸) or the Stability sequence (see page 57 ◂).

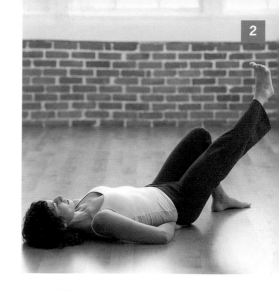

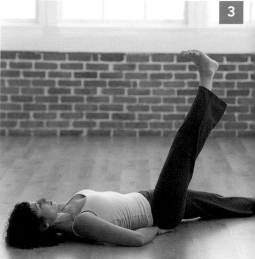

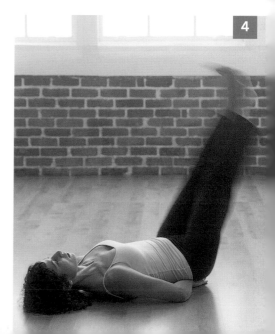

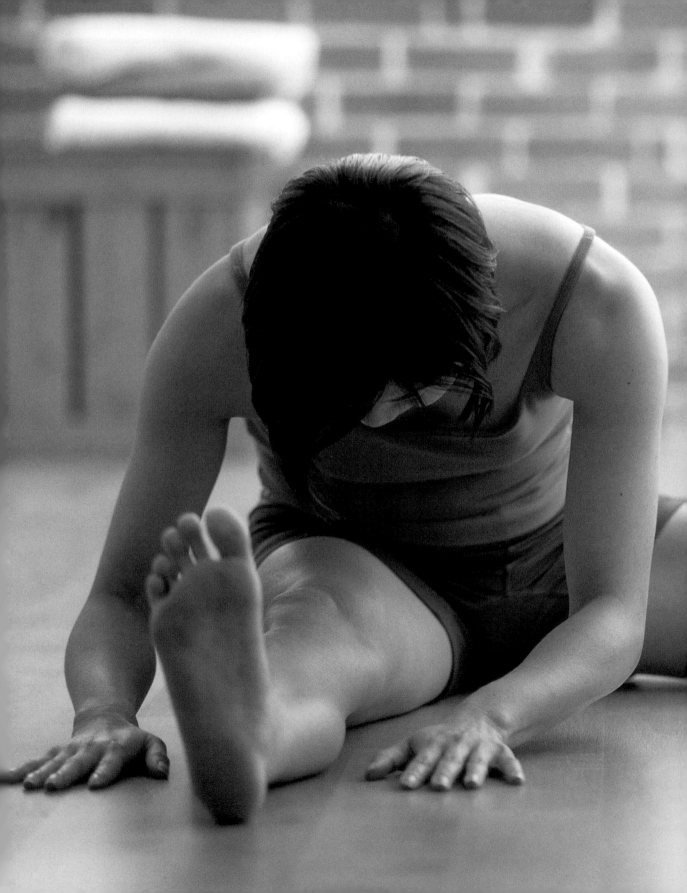

revival

The repetitive exercises of most workouts build strength, but they can also shorten and tighten your muscles, decreasing range of motion and inhibiting your performance. That's why flexibility is a vital component of fitness. Post-workout stretches lengthen your muscles and soothe your nervous system. And they help keep your body as supple as it is powerful.

key benefits

▶ Increases flexibility and range of motion

▶ Lengthens muscles

▶ Helps avoid post-workout soreness

stay supple

At the end of a workout, perform this rewarding ritual of yoga poses to help keep your muscles supple and ease your mind back into the world.

1 reclining hip hug

Lying on your back, bring your right knee to your chest and wrap your hands around your leg. Gently pull your thigh towards your chest. Hold for a few breaths. Then rest your right arm on your inner right thigh and your left hand on your left hip and rotate your right leg out towards the floor, keeping it bent. Hold for a few breaths. Release. Repeat on the other side.

2 forward bend

Sit with your legs extended, knees straight but not locked, feet flexed but not rigid. (If it's difficult to sit up straight in this position, sit on the edge of a firm pillow or folded blanket, as shown). Then lift your hands overhead shoulder-width apart and inhale, lengthening your back. Exhaling, fold forwards from your hips, grasp both legs or feet (whichever you can reach comfortably), and let your head and shoulders hang. Hold for a minute, releasing and sitting up on an inhalation.

3 seated and revolved wide angle

For the Seated Wide Angle pose, sit with your legs spread wide, feet pointed upwards. (If it's an effort to sit upright, you can sit on a firm pillow or folded blanket.) Place your hands on the floor between your legs. To increase the intensity, walk your hands forwards on the floor. Try not to drop your head or let your back round as you hold the pose for a minute.

To move into Revolved Wide Angle, turn your chest and hips to face your right foot. Place your palms on the floor on either side of your right leg, inhale and elongate your spine. Exhaling, slowly walk your hands towards your right foot. Lower your chest towards your leg; try to keep your left hip on the ground. Hold for 30 seconds. Release. Repeat facing the other leg.

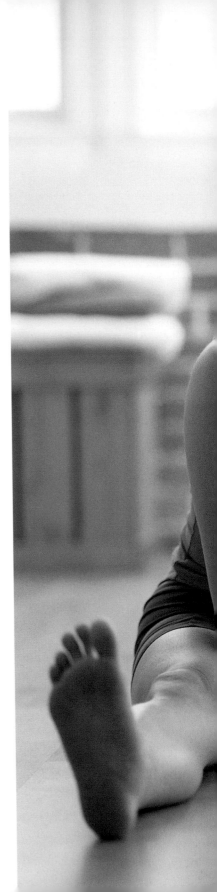

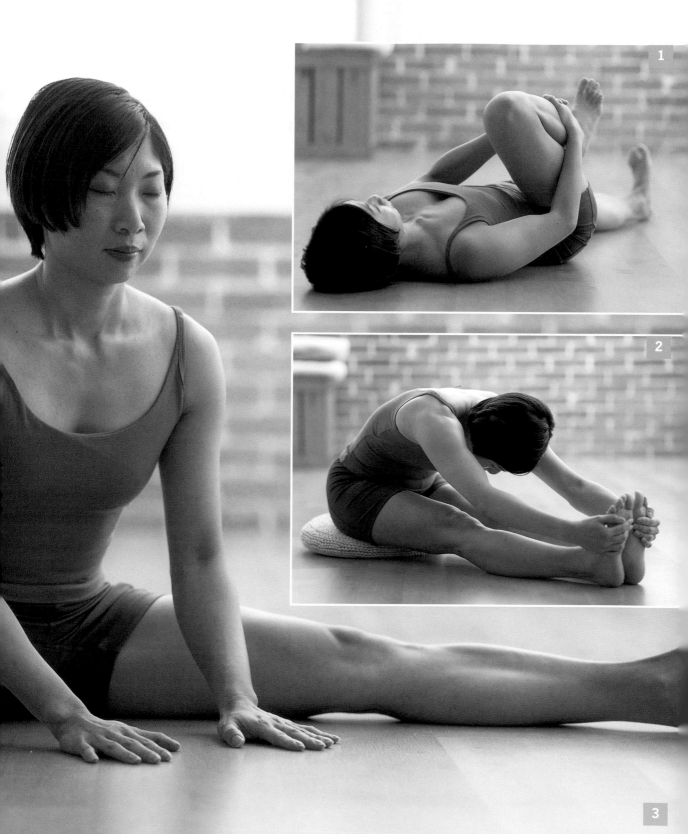

1

2

3

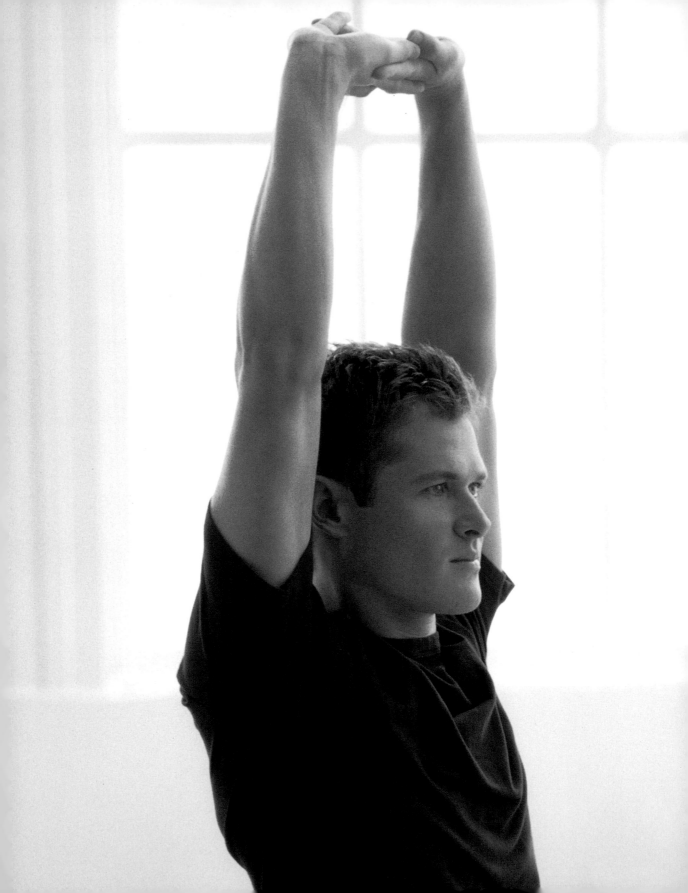

renewal

Sitting at a desk for long periods creates discomfort and strain that make it difficult to do your job well. Yoga can help alleviate everyday stresses, increasing wellbeing and efficiency. A yoga break at work lessens the chances of developing a repetitive-strain injury and may mean a more productive and enjoyable day.

key benefits

► Decreases stress and increases concentration

► Reduces the risk of repetitive-strain injury

► Helps you work more productively

renewal

at-work workout

These simple stretches will help elevate your energy and loosen upper-body tension built up by too much time at your desk. And you can do them from your office chair.

1 folding leaf

Place your palms on the front edge of your desk, shoulder-width apart. Slide your chair back until your back and arms are fully extended and your head is down. Hold for four breaths, then release your hands and let your arms hang, bringing your chest to (or towards) your thighs. Relax for up to a minute, then sit up.

2 reach for the sky

Interlace your fingers and lift your hands overhead. Gently turn your palms towards the ceiling, stopping at any sign of wrist discomfort. If it's more comfortable, turn your palms down. Bring your shoulders back and down. Extend your hands up, lengthening your body with each breath. Hold and stretch upwards for several breaths.

3 seated crescent moon

Place your left hand on the seat of your chair and lift your right arm overhead. Exhaling, press your hips downwards to ground them, then inhale and stretch your right side by pressing up into your right hand and arching to the left. To counter a tendency to roll forwards, gaze upwards and raise your chest towards the ceiling. Hold for 4–8 breaths; inhale as you release and repeat on the other side.

4 chair twist

Sitting sideways on an armless chair with your left hip against the back, inhale and lengthen your spine. Exhale and gently rotate to the left, working from the base of your spine upwards, and grasp both sides of the chair back. With each inhalation, elongate your spine; with each exhalation, gently increase your rotation. Visualise this twist as wringing tension from your mind as well as from your body. Hold for about 30 seconds; release gently, starting from your shoulders, then repeat, twisting to the other side.

Work Savvy
- Rather than relying on caffeine, eliminate tiredness and raise concentration levels at work with essential oils: peppermint, to refresh and stimulate; lemon, to uplift and enliven; and sweet orange, to balance and lift moods. Use any of these oils in a diffuser, or sprinkle a little oil on a tissue and keep it at your desk. (When using undiluted essential oils, avoid any direct contact with the skin.)
- "Palming" your eyes can help ease eye strain. Rub your hands together briskly, then lightly press them to your closed eyes with your fingers pointing upwards. Visualise comfort emanating from them, and let the warmth soothe your eyes.

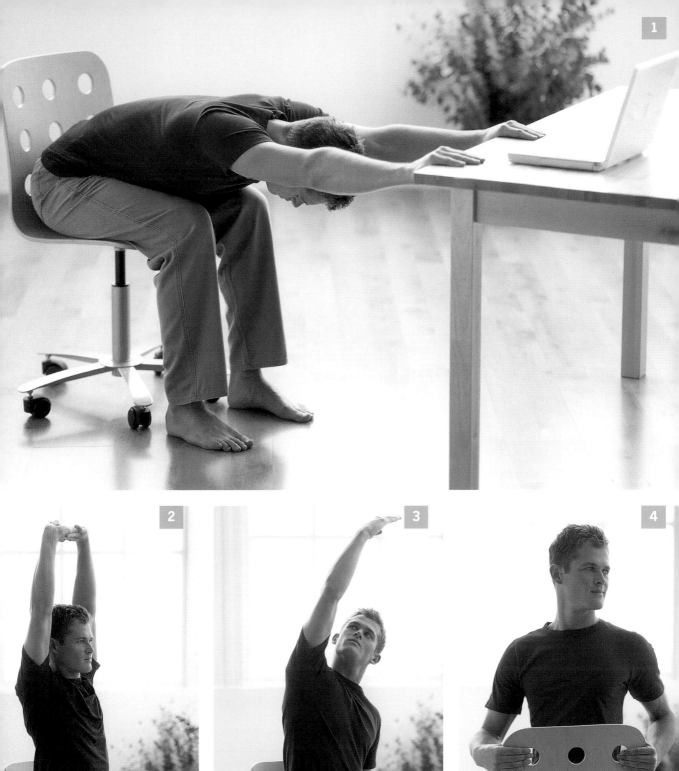

harmony

Premenstrual syndrome may create disharmony in your body and thoughts, but yoga practice can help correct that imbalance. Relaxation poses calm your mind and help diminish irritability, gentle stretches aid relaxation, and mild inversions may relieve bloating. So take some quiet time to restore your natural tranquillity.

key benefits

- ▶ Helps relieve premenstrual symptoms
- ▶ Helps reduce bloating
- ▶ Eases lower-body muscle tension

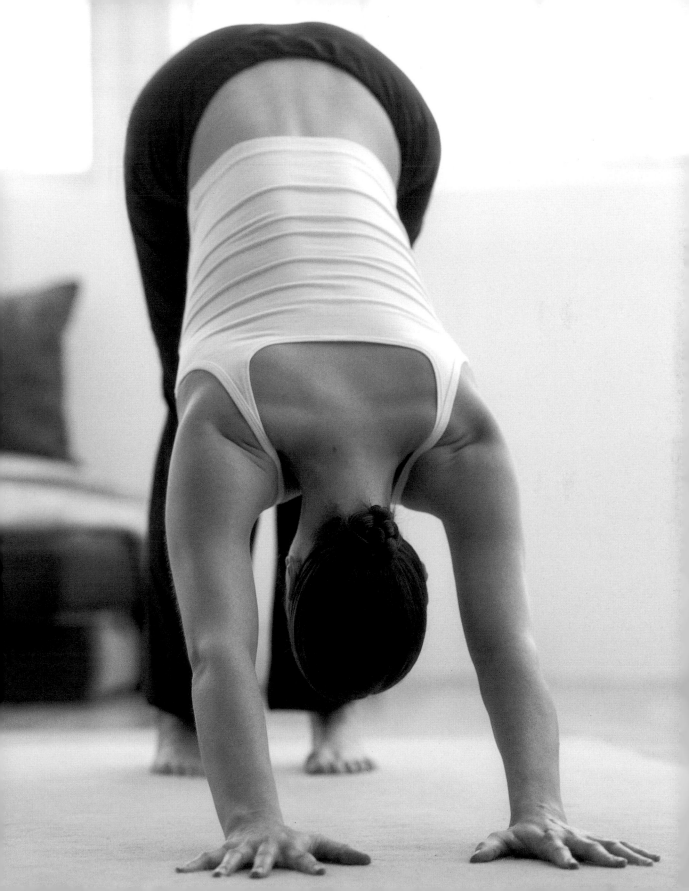

ease your cycle

Draw yourself inwards and tune into your body with these poses designed to help smooth the physical and mental rough edges that can arise from PMS.

Aromatherapy Menstrual TLC
- To help ease mood swings, scent your room using a spray-mister filled with 10 drops of bergamot, lavender or geranium essential oil and 120 ml of water.
- To help relieve fluid retention, add 5 drops of patchouli or rosemary essential oil to 2 teaspoons of your carrier oil of choice (such as sweet almond, grapeseed or jojoba) and massage your abdomen.
- To help quiet menstrual cramps, add 5 drops of chamomile or 2 drops of clary sage essential oil to a bowl of cool water, wet a towel in the bowl and put it on your abdomen for ten minutes.

1 downward dog

Begin on your hands and knees (the Table position) with your hands shoulder-width apart, your fingers spread wide, and your middle fingers pointing forwards. With your feet hip-width apart, lift your hips and press through your arms and hands out to your fingertips. To protect your wrists, try to keep the pressure at the base of your index finger and thumb. Continue to press your hips upwards and your chest towards your feet, letting your heels sink towards the floor. Hold for 4–10 breaths, then relax back down into the Table position.

2 camel

Kneel with your knees and feet hip-width apart. Place your hands on your hips with your thumbs against your lower back; exhale, tighten your buttocks and move your hips forwards. Then inhale and arch your upper back without dropping your head. (If you're comfortable, you can try to bring your hands to your heels, one at a time, letting your head hang back.) Hold for several breaths, then lift your head and roll forwards, one shoulder at a time, to release.

3 wide angle at wall

Sitting sideways along a wall with your knees bent, slowly turn and lower your back to the floor, raising your legs against the wall at the same time. Make sure your lower back is in contact with the floor. Separate your legs into a wide V shape and rest your arms (palms up) on the floor a comfortable distance from your body. Hold for 1–5 minutes, then release by letting your knees sink to your chest.

4 side child pose

Roll onto your right side with your knees close to your chest. Use your right arm to cushion your head with your left arm resting comfortably on your legs. Rest in this pose for a minute, observing the sensations of comfort and wellbeing in your body and mind.

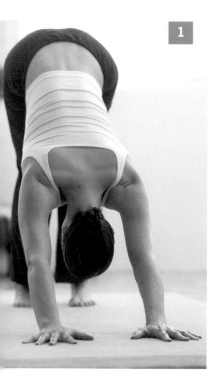

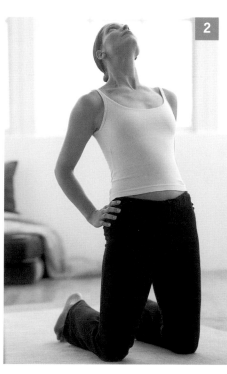

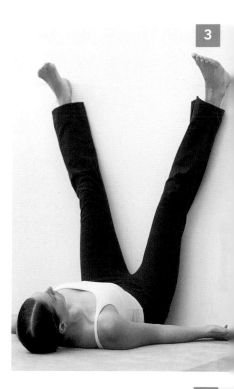

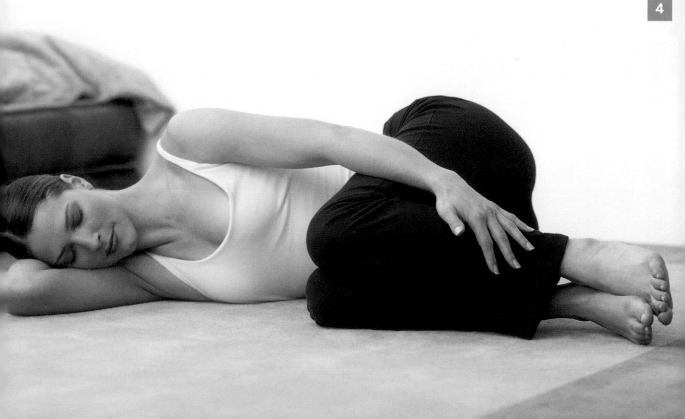

pair against PMS

When premenstrual syndrome has you feeling blue or uncomfortable, doing yoga with a friend may be just the thing to reduce discomfort and cheer you up. Partner variations lessen the effort required of your arms and back. This support can allow you to hold the poses longer than you might on your own, providing a greater benefit.

Downward Dog is a remarkably efficient pose for harmonising the body. It stretches and strengthens your arms, legs and back all at once, while also providing a partial inversion.

The Stone and Sky pose can be emotionally as well as physically comforting: the warmth of another body against yours can calm frayed emotions and ease sore muscles.

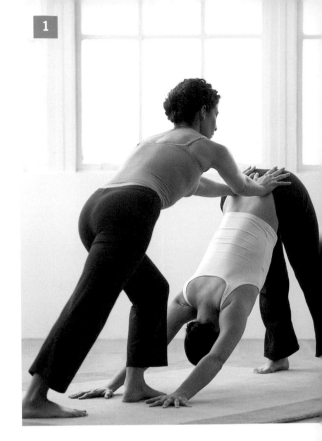

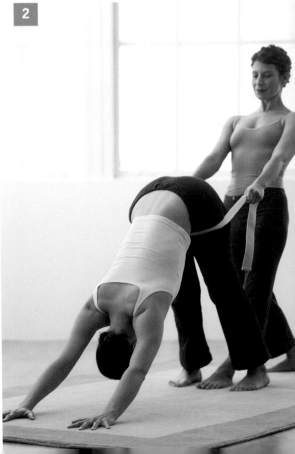

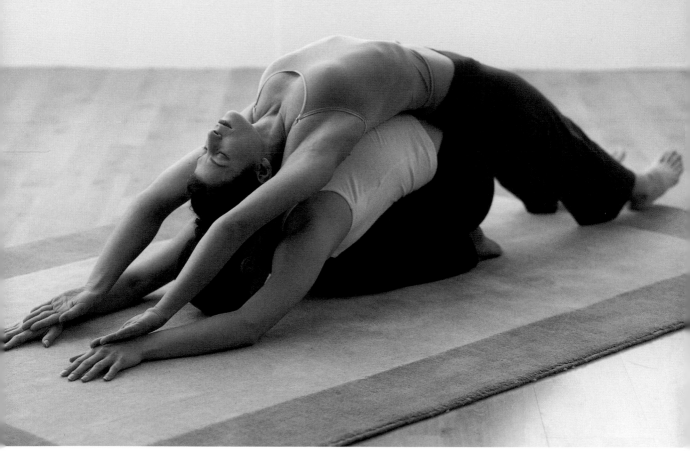

1 rising downward dog

As you move into the Downward Dog pose (page 72 ◄), have your partner stand at your head, placing one of her feet between your hands and the other a comfortable distance behind her. She should then put both hands on your lower back and press firmly with straight arms up towards your tailbone, keeping her spine erect and leaning forward as much as you indicate feels comfortable. Hold for a few minutes, then relax into the Child pose (page 87 ►).

2 lifted downward dog

In this variation of Downward Dog, ask your partner to stand at your feet and slip a yoga strap or a smooth belt around your upper thighs, holding the strap at a point that allows her to keep her arms straight. Ask her to place one of her feet between yours and the other a comfortable distance back. Ask her then to lean back gently so that the pull of the strap creates a pleasant release in your lower back while lessening the effort of your arms. Hold for a few minutes, then sink into Child.

3 stone and sky

Resting in Child with your hands extended forwards, ask your partner to face away from you, sit lightly on your hips and then slowly extend her legs, reclining into a backbend along your back. Then ask your partner to extend her arms overhead. If your hands are close, link them and breathe together, staying in this position for a minute or two.

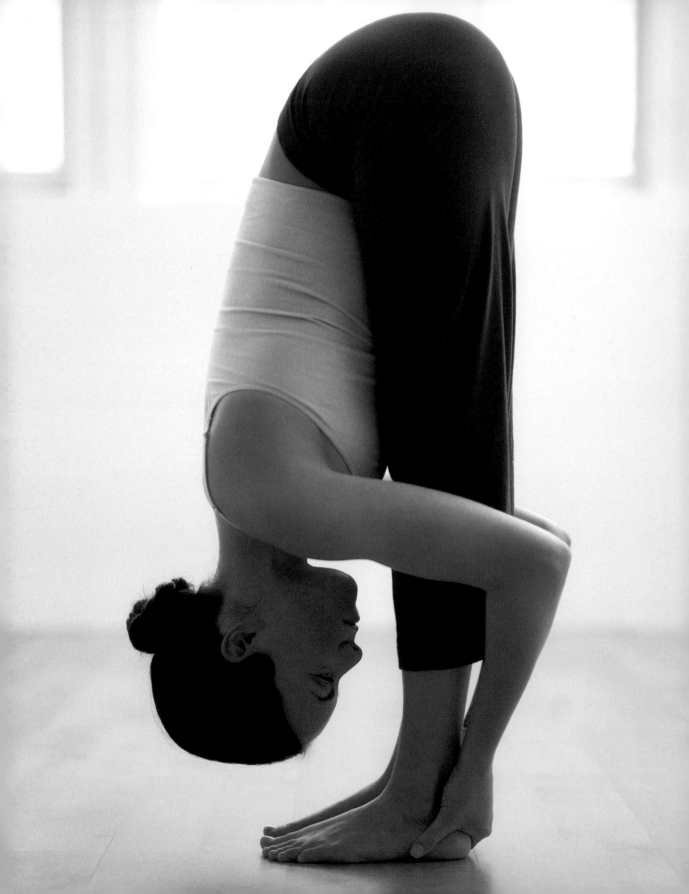

freedom

If lower-back tension has your body in knots and your mind in a fog, yoga may offer a solution. Gentle poses massage your lower back and abdominal organs, help increase your range of motion, and strengthen core muscles. Regular, gentle practice can work both to ease discomfort and transform your body.

key benefits

► Increases flexibility in back and hips

► Alleviates tension in lower back

► Helps clear your mind

focus on your back

This sequence is designed to relieve back tension and improve flexibility. While the focus here is on your body, don't be surprised if your head feels clearer as a bonus.

1 pelvic tilt

Lie on your back with your hands on the floor beside your hips, your knees bent and your feet on the floor hip-width apart. Inhale, arching your lower back and pressing your tailbone down, then exhale, flattening your lower back down to the floor. Continue practising for 4–10 breaths, arching with each inhalation and flattening with each exhalation, gently relaxing your lower back.

2 lying twist

With legs together and knees bent, extend your arms out from your shoulders along the floor, palms down. Lower your bent legs towards the floor on your left, gazing either upwards or, if comfort allows, to your right. If your left hand reaches comfortably, place it on your knees to add a little extra weight. Hold for ten breaths, inhale as you bring your legs back to centre, then repeat on your right side.

3 wind-relieving pose

Lift your knees to your chest, then wrap your arms around your legs. Inhale deeply and hold your breath as you lift your chest towards your knees. Rock – from side to side or from head to hips – so the weight of your body massages your back. Exhale quickly and forcefully through your mouth as you drop your limbs to the floor. Relax.

4 standing forward bend

Stand with your feet together and your palms together in front of your heart. Inhale and extend your hands forwards, palms facing down, arms shoulder-width apart and parallel to the floor, then raise them overhead. Keeping your arms alongside your ears, exhale and fold forwards from your hips, letting arms and head hang. To ease the stretch, bend your knees slightly. To intensify it, grasp your legs or heels, coaxing your head towards your feet (bottom photo). Hold for 30–60 seconds, then bend your knees and roll up on an inhalation.

Back to Basics

- High-heeled shoes raise the back of your pelvis as well as your heels, increasing the arch of your lumbar spine (lower back). If you have lower back discomfort, try wearing flat or low-heeled shoes.
- At your desk, use a chair with lumbar support and try to stand up and move around at least once each hour. Also try the Renewal sequence shown on pages 68–69 ◄.
- When lifting heavy or bulky objects, bend and lift with your legs and try to keep your back straight.

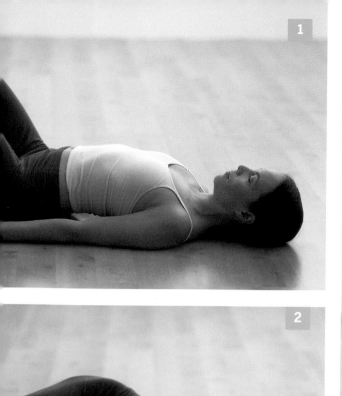

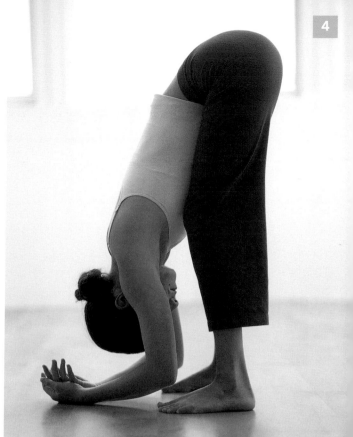

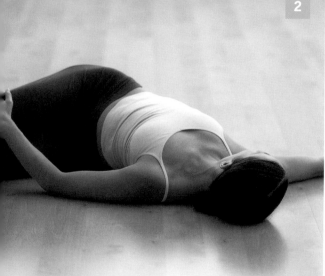

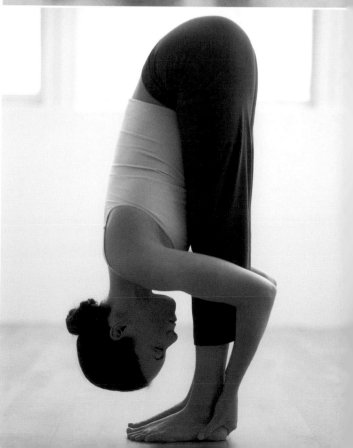

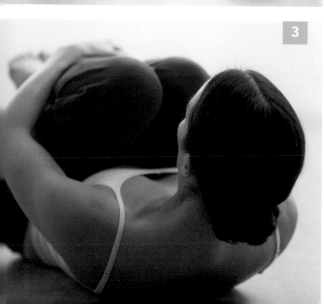

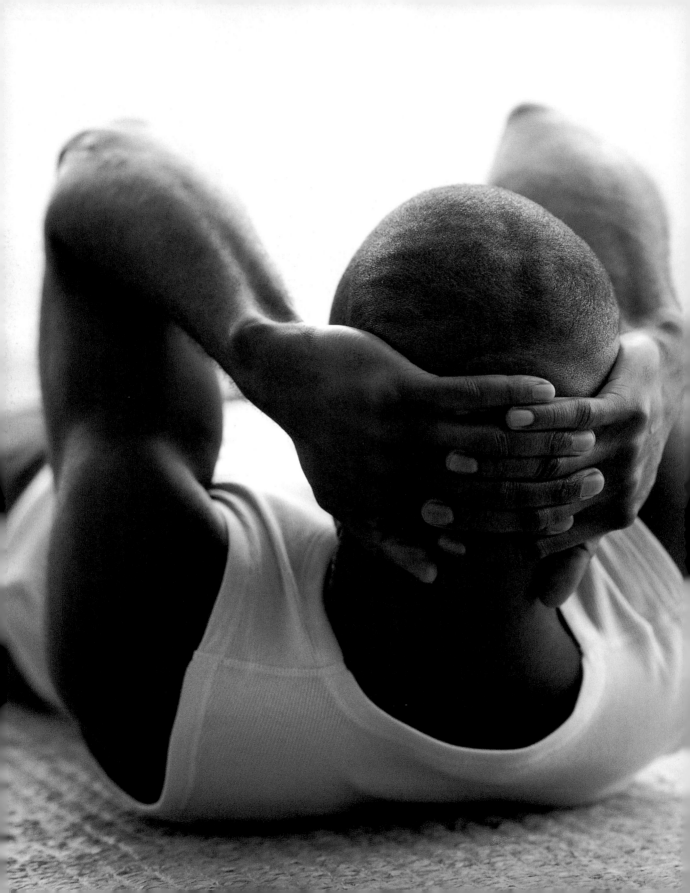

energy

Ancient yogis believed that practising inversions promised immortality. That might be a bit optimistic, but inversions definitely do a body good. These yoga poses can stimulate your endocrine system, which helps regulate your metabolism. Metabolic processes transform nutrients into energy, which sustains life. So turn yourself upside down and give your life a lift.

key benefits

► Boosts immune function

► Strengthens abdominal and back muscles

► Helps balance your metabolism

rev up your metabolism

Your metabolism can have a profound impact on both your weight and energy. If you think yours might be on the sluggish side, add inversions to your yoga practice.

Take Note
- It is essential to do the Fish pose after Candle, as it acts as a balancing counterpose.
- Full inversions like the Candle pose are not always beneficial. If you're menstruating; have recently had dental work; or have a hiatal hernia, uncontrolled high blood pressure, headache, or back, head or neck injuries, substitute Restful Inversion (see page 87 ▶) or Wide Angle at Wall (see page 72 ◀).
- Your thyroid gland, a crucial part of the endocrine system, helps regulate your body's metabolic processes. It lies at the base of your throat, so the compression in this sequence (poses 1–4) can help massage and tone your thyroid.

1 lifted cradle

Throughout this pose, your arms do the work and your neck muscles remain passive. Lying on your back, interlace your fingers and cradle the back of your head, bringing your arms up alongside your ears. With your hands, gently raise your head and lift it away from your shoulders, lengthening the back of your neck, then continue to lift so your chin moves towards your chest. Hold for 4–6 breaths and release.

2 bridge

Lie on your back, bend your knees, and put your feet hip-width apart on the floor. As you inhale, press your palms down on the floor next to your hips and lift your hips towards the ceiling. Put your hands on your lower back for support; keep your knees directly above your heels. Hold for 4–10 breaths. On an exhalation, release your hands to the floor and slowly roll your back down, from neck to tailbone.

3 candle

Lying on the floor, press your palms down beside your hips, lift your legs towards the ceiling and roll your hips off the floor; use your hands to support your back. Lift your legs as upright as comfort allows. Hold this position for two minutes, bending your knees if you want to rest. To come out of the pose, first lower your legs overhead (towards the floor), placing your palms on the floor for support. Then slowly roll down, bending your knees if you need to rest your back.

4 fish

Place your palms against the sides of your outer thighs. Without moving your arms, press your elbows into the floor and lift your head and chest to look at your feet. Arch your chest and lower the top of your head back and down to the floor. Balance your weight between buttocks, arms and head. Hold for 4–10 breaths. To release, press down with your arms as you lift your head and roll down.

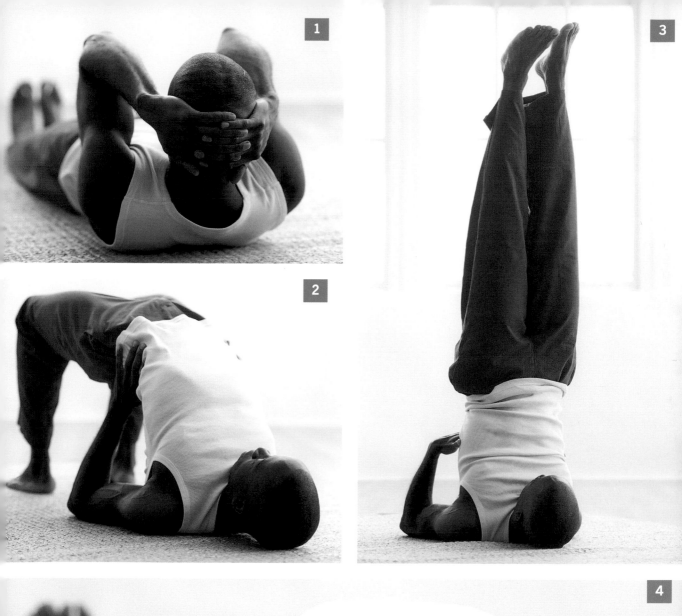
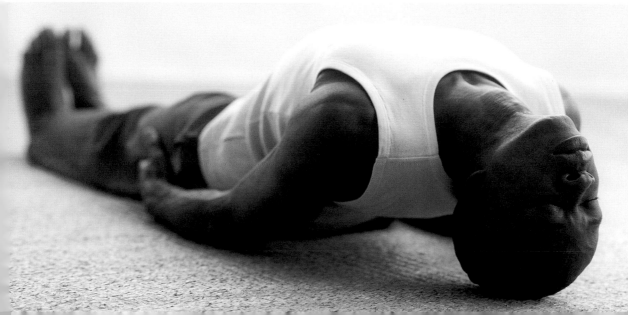

health

You know it when you see and feel it: the radiant glow of health. Whether you're fighting off a cold or just hoping to maximise wellbeing, yoga can aid your immune system. By stimulating your lymphatic and endocrine systems and soothing your nervous system, regular yoga practice can help keep you glowing.

key benefits

▸ Helps boost immunity

▸ Calms the nervous system

▸ Instils a sense of wellbeing

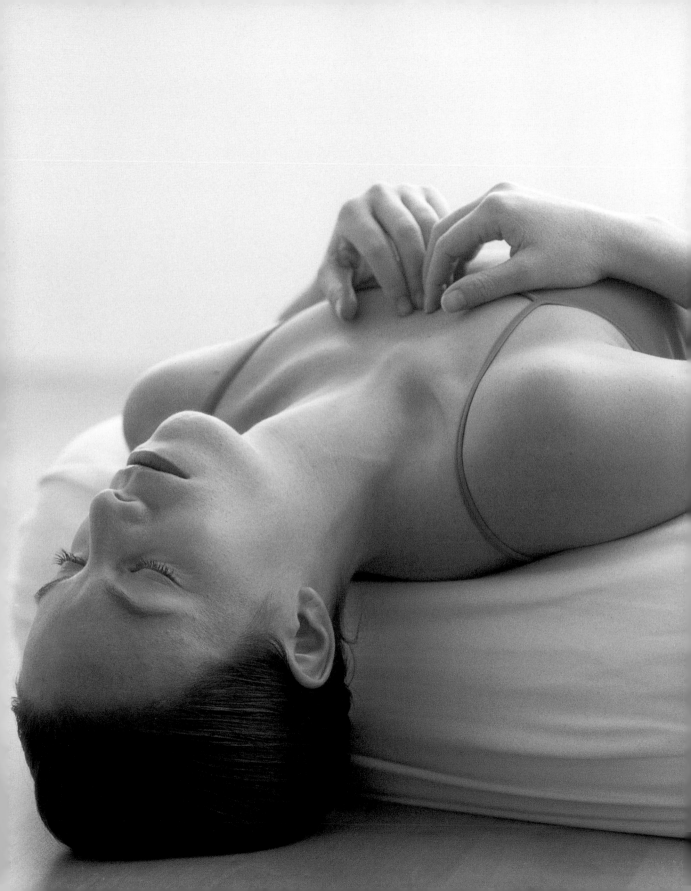

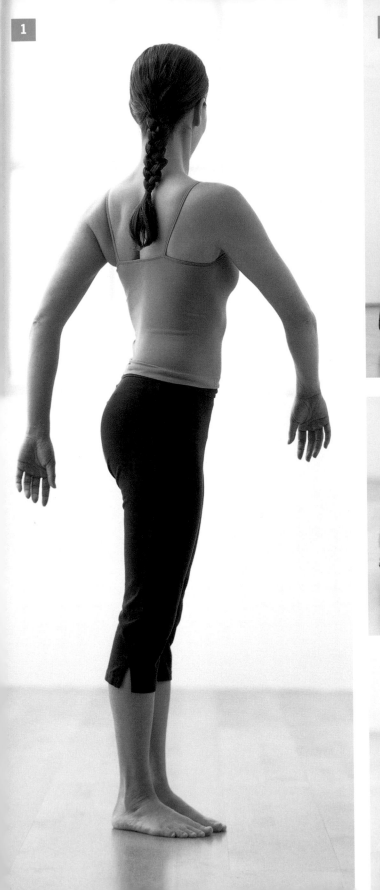

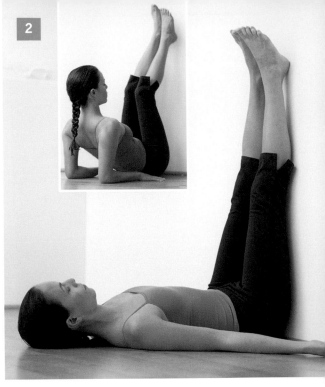

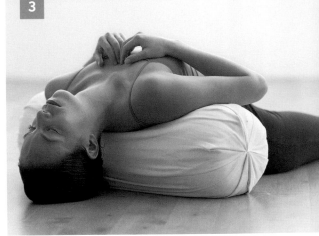

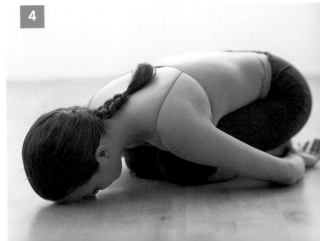

boost your resistance

These poses target key body hot spots, such as the lymph and thymus glands, to aid your immune system, heighten awareness and foster feelings of tranquillity.

1 swinging twist

Standing with your feet together and your arms hanging loose, begin to twist your torso gently from side to side, allowing your arms to swing and bump lightly against your body. Gradually increase speed so that the force of the swings lifts your arms away from your body. Continue for a minute or two to stimulate the lymph glands in your underarms; then stand and rest in the Mountain pose (page 30 ◄).

2 restful inversion

Sitting sideways next to a wall with knees bent, turn your back away from the wall, raising your legs against the wall (see inset). Lower your back to the floor while keeping your hips in contact with the floor. Rest your arms on the floor, palms up. Hold for 1–5 minutes, as comfort allows. If you need to rest, bend your knees. To come out of this pose, let your knees sink towards your chest and roll to one side.

3 supported fish

Place a bolster or a rolled-up blanket on the floor and lie back so that it supports your upper back, while the back of the crown of your head touches the floor. Gently drum your fingertips on your breastbone (the centre of your chest) to stimulate your thymus gland, an important regulator in your immune system. Hold for one minute, then use your arms to raise yourself up into a sitting position.

4 child

From a kneeling position, sit back on your heels, then lean forwards and bring your chest towards your knees and your forehead towards the floor. If your forehead does not rest on the floor, let your head hang or rest it on a firm pillow. Place your hands alongside your feet, palms up, and relax, enjoying the gentle stretch of your lower back and hips. Try to quieten your thoughts and draw your awareness inwards. Hold for a minute or two, then inhale as you rise up to release.

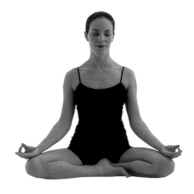

Skull Shining Breath

Kapalabhati, the Skull Shining Breath, is an energising and purifying practice of rapid, forceful diaphragmatic exhalations and automatic, passive inhalations. Sitting comfortably with your mouth closed, snap your abdomen inwards to exhale, and relax your abdomen to inhale. Begin with three rounds of 20 exhalations, increasing over time to 100 exhalations. At the end of each round, exhale completely, then inhale, filling your lungs fully, and finally exhale as slowly as you can. Rest briefly after each round.

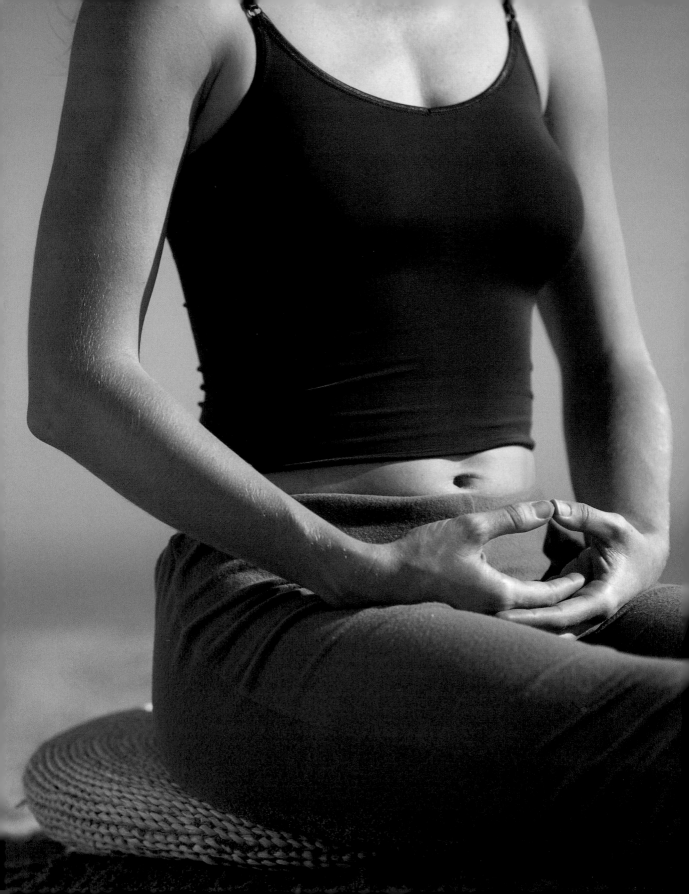

purity

Purity is one of the qualities yogis cultivate to achieve health and harmony. One way to accomplish this is to consciously undertake practices that detoxify the body. While it's common to think of yoga poses as stretches, many also provide compression that massages your internal organs, helping to keep you clean and clear.

key benefits

▶ Helps detoxify your system

▶ Clears your mind

▶ Massages vital internal organs

detox and clear

These poses can be practised just about anywhere, although a tranquil outdoor setting – such as a beach or garden – fosters a sense of connection to nature.

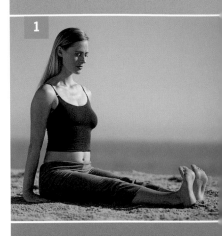

1 staff

Sit with your legs extended, knees straight but not locked, and feet flexed. Place your palms on the ground beside your hips, fingers pointing towards your toes. (If it's difficult to sit straight, sit on a firm pillow or folded blanket.) Hold for ten breaths.

2 head to knee

Bending your left leg, place the sole of your left foot against your right inner thigh as close to your hips as comfort allows without drawing your left hip backwards. Drop your left knee towards the ground. Lift your arms overhead and inhale, elongating your spine. Exhale, folding forwards from your hips. Align the centre of your chest with the centre of your right leg, grasp your right leg or foot, and let your head hang. Hold for a minute. Inhale as you rise up. Repeat on the other side.

3 half spinal twist

Place your left foot on the right side of your right calf. Inhale and lengthen your spine; exhale and turn towards your left. Bring your left hand to the ground behind your back for support and place your right arm on the left side of your left leg for leverage as you twist. Look over your left shoulder. Hold for 30 seconds. Untwist and repeat on the other side.

4 half bow

Lying face forwards, bend your right leg and reach back with your right hand to grasp your ankle (for a greater challenge, try using your left hand). Place your resting forearm on the ground in front of your chest. With your back arm straight and hips flat, lift your head, neck and chest as you press your heel away from your back into your hand and lift your thigh. Hold for 4–10 breaths. Release and repeat on the other side.

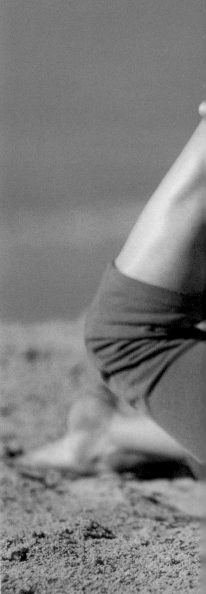

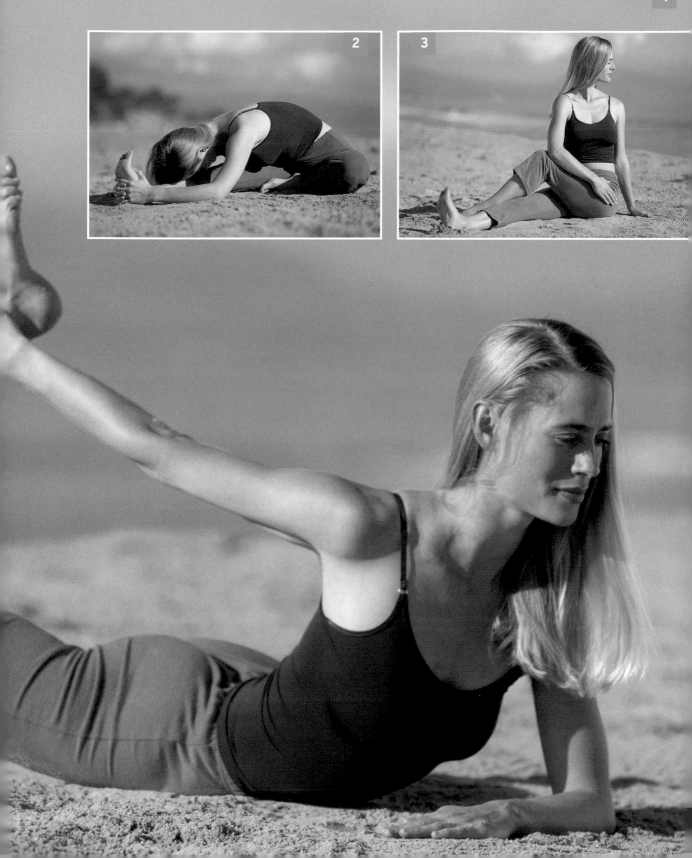

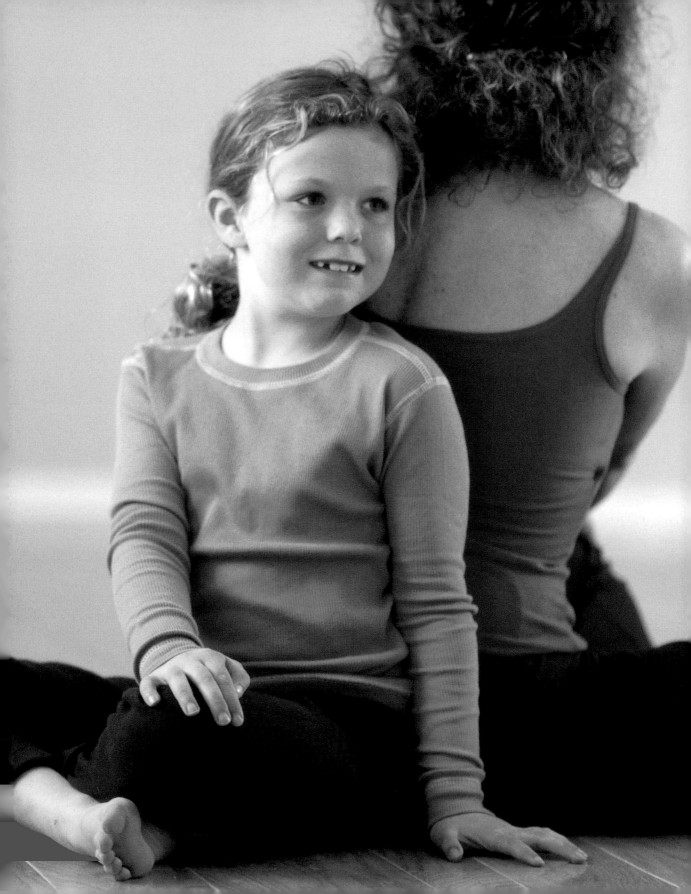

comfort

A sanctuary is a place of safety and peace, a place to
cast aside cares and replenish yourself. It's also a state
of mind. You can create a sanctuary anywhere by
finding your calm centre and nurturing yourself with
poses that release energy trapped in tight muscles. Then
use that energy to maintain your serenity and vitality.

key benefits

- ▶ Releases tension trapped in muscles
- ▶ Boosts vigour
- ▶ Restores tranquillity

comfort

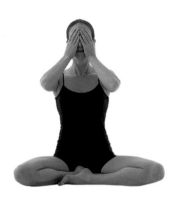

Humming Bee Breath
Brahmari, the Humming Bee Breath, clarifies and calms with a pleasing sound vibration and is a breathing practice enjoyed by children as well as adults. Place your hands over your eyes and use your thumbs to close your ears. Inhale deeply, then exhale slowly through your nostrils, humming high in the back of your mouth so the sound vibrates into your soft palate. Practise this for 3–7 breaths, then release, close your eyes and observe the quiet.

find stillness

Close the door on the rest of the world – literally and figuratively. Enrich body and soul with deep, regular breathing, and take comfort in these yoga poses.

1 lifting wings

Standing with your feet hip-width apart, interlace your hands behind your back, palms up. Fold forwards, bringing your chest towards your legs and pressing your hands away from your back. (Bend your knees if you want to lessen the intensity in your legs and increase it in your shoulders.) Hold for 8–10 breaths, then release.

2 folding wings

Sitting cross-legged, elongate your spine, interlace your fingers and put your hands on the back of your head. Inhaling, press your elbows back without pressing on your head, opening your shoulders. Exhale as you fold your arms in towards your ears, lengthen the back of your neck and bring your chin towards your chest. Repeat for four breaths, inhaling as you open up your elbows, exhaling as you pull them in.

3 rainbow

From a comfortable seated position, place your right hand on the floor at your right. Lift your left hand up with your thumb facing back. Inhale and stretch upwards, then exhale and arch to the right. Let your right arm bend, reach your left hand to the right, and look forwards or slightly upwards. Keep your chest up and hold the pose for 4–8 breaths, inhaling as you straighten up. Repeat on the other side.

4 yogic seal

Sitting comfortably, bring your hands behind your back and gently grasp the wrist of your dominant hand with your other hand. Inhale and elongate your spine, then exhale as you fold forwards from your hips. Keep your hands relaxed against your back. Let your head hang towards, or rest against, the floor. If your head is uncomfortable, place a firm pillow under it. Direct your mind to an inner place of stillness. Hold for 30–60 seconds, then slowly sit up on an inhalation.

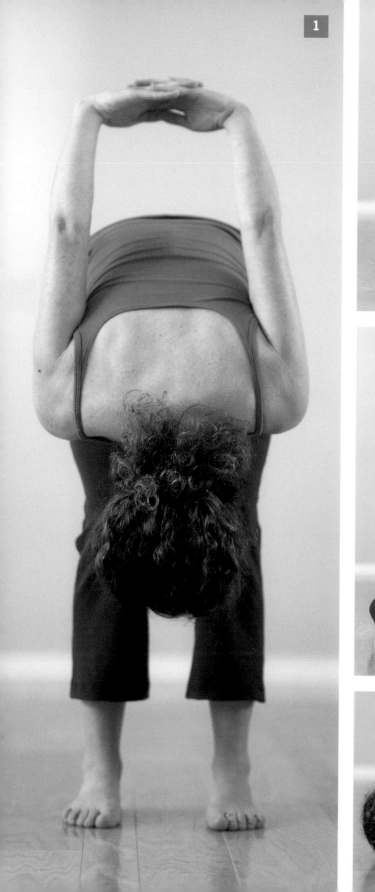

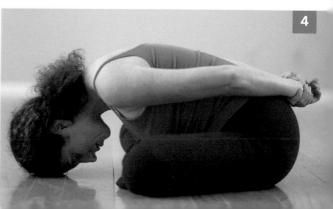

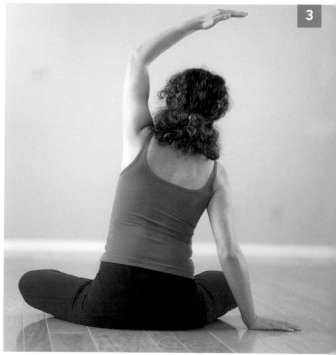

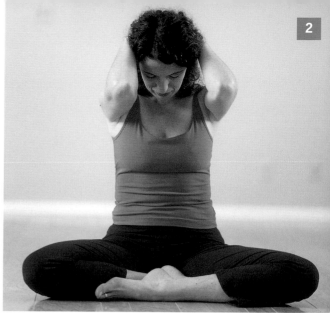

comfort

youthful yoga

Doing poses together is a marvellous way to bond with your child. Practice helps kids explore the body's possibilities – and appreciate the joys of stillness.

Kidding Around
- It's natural for children to explore the constantly changing possibilities of their bodies. And while kids love to stretch their bodies, their minds tend to jump around. To keep focused as you practise, try counting together, talking about what's happening with your bodies, or practising the Humming Bee Breath (page 94 ◄).
- This sequence begins in motion and slows into a shared repose, a quieter experience that can help a child discover the pleasure and comfort that stillness can offer.

1 rocking seat

Sit back-to-back with your partner, legs straight forwards and arms relaxed. Inhale and lengthen your back, then exhale and lean forwards, placing your hands on your legs or feet. Ask your partner to follow you, lying against your back with her arms relaxed forwards or raised overhead. Hold for several breaths, then rise to centre together on an inhalation. Repeat, reversing roles, so your partner leans forwards and you backwards. (If you are practising this pose with a child, make sure that you don't lean back too heavily.)

2 braided rope

Sitting cross-legged back to back with your partner, inhale together as you elongate your spines. Placing your right hand on your left knee and your left hand on the floor to your left (with your partner doing the same), exhale as you each turn to your own left, keeping your backs together as you both twist. Hold for several breaths, then return to the centre and repeat, rotating to the right this time.

3 sharing breath

Sit cross-legged either on the floor or sharing a pillow with your back against your partner's. Place your hands on your knees or lap and close your eyes as your partner does the same. Focus on each other's breathing and see if you can synchronise your breaths. Try to concentrate completely on breathing. If you notice your mind wandering, just bring it back to your breath. Sit quietly and breathe together for as long as it feels comfortable to both of you.

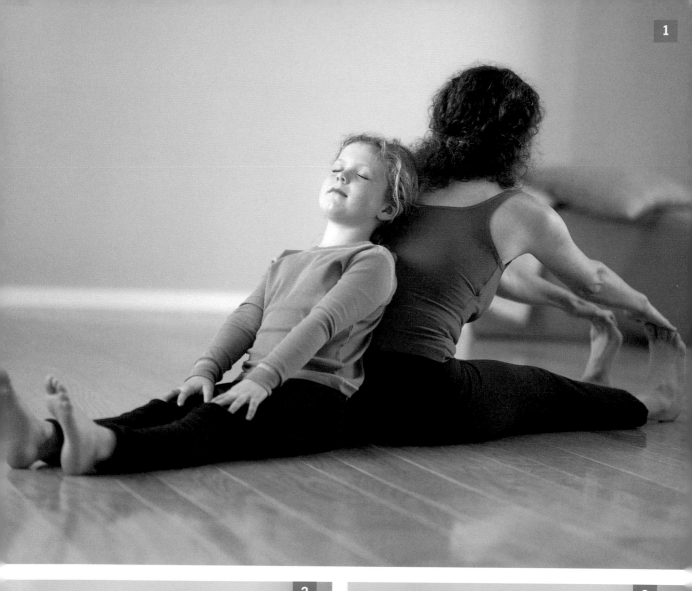

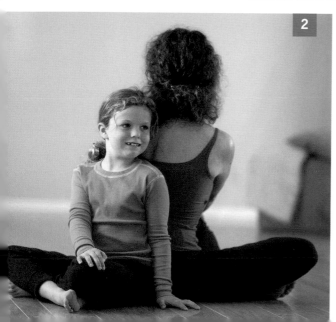

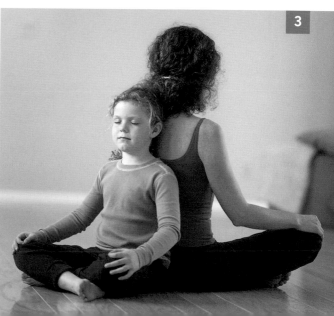

peace

Sleep is a unique state of consciousness, a vital and restorative period for body, mind and soul. Finding your way to that state, though, can sometimes be a challenge. Take time at night for relaxation and release. Use breathing and meditation practices to help slow and calm your mind, guiding you to soothing slumber.

key benefits

- ▶ Helps you let go of the day's cares
- ▶ Relaxes your body
- ▶ Prepares you for a peaceful night's rest

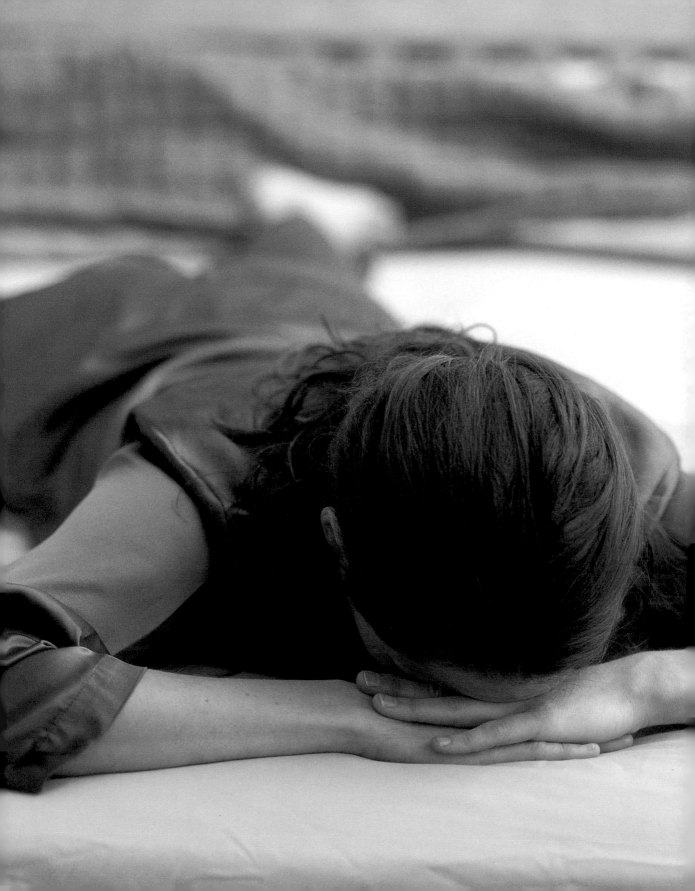

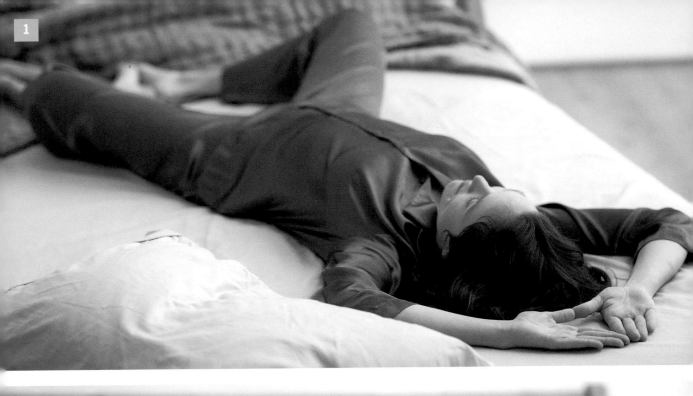

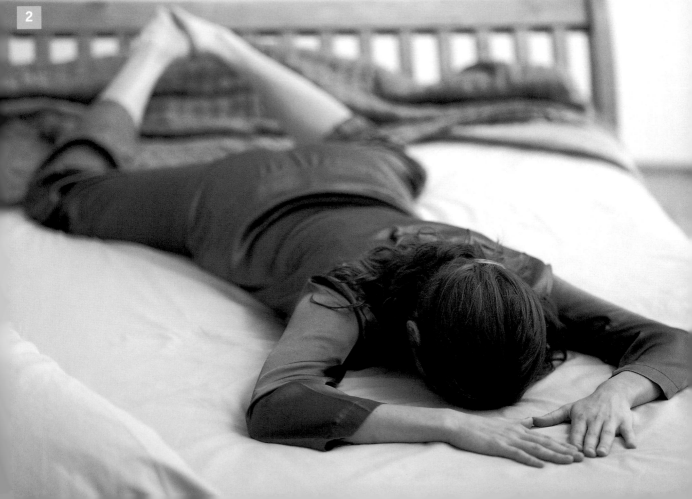

come to rest

These yoga poses release your mind's preoccupations and your body's tensions, helping to guide you towards deep relaxation and, eventually, blissful sleep.

1 corpse and upward triple diamond

Lying flat on your back with legs straight but relaxed and your feet shoulder-width apart (not pictured), rest your arms at a comfortable distance from your body, palms up. Close your eyes. Scan your body mentally from head to toe. As you observe tension in any area of your body, visualise your breath moving in and out of that spot, dissolving the tension. Relax in this pose for 1–5 minutes.

Bring the soles of your feet together and let your knees sink to the sides (see photo). Raise your arms overhead with palms up and your thumbs and index fingers together. Let the weight of your arms and legs sink downwards, bringing release to your hips and shoulders. As your body relaxes for a minute or so, feel your mind begin to empty.

2 downward triple diamond and crocodile

Lying face down, lift your arms overhead and bring your thumbs and index fingers together, palms down. Bend your knees, then slide them apart and bring the soles of your feet together (see photo). Relax your hips. For greater intensity, you might gently press your feet downwards. Hold for ten breaths, drawing your mind deeply inwards. Lift your feet and bring your legs together to release.

Straighten your legs and turn your feet outwards, moving your legs far enough apart for this to be comfortable (see page 99 ◄). Place your right hand in front of your face, palm down; place your left hand on top of your right; and rest your forehead on your hands. Rest for 1–5 minutes, focusing on your breathing and enjoying the peace.

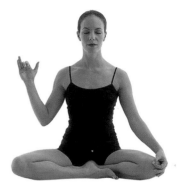

Alternate Nostril Breathing
Nadi suddhi, Alternate Nostril Breathing, is superb for balancing the subtler energies of the body and mind before meditation or sleep. Fold the index and middle fingers of your right hand into your palm (if it's comfortable), then close your right nostril with your thumb, exhaling through the left nostril. Inhale through the left nostril, then close it with your ring and little fingers, releasing your thumb and exhaling through your right nostril. Continue the pattern (exhale-inhale-switch) for 1–5 minutes.

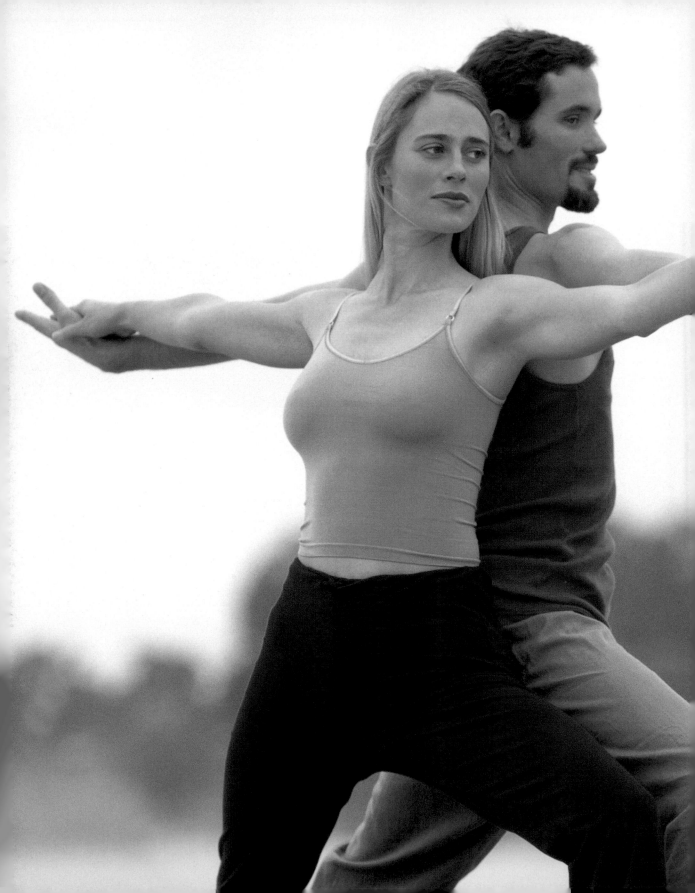

union

The definition of the word *yoga* is "union". Feeling
at one with yourself – and with all things – is the
ultimate goal in yoga. Individual practice fosters a
feeling of groundedness, heightens self-awareness, and
hones both physical and mental control. Practising yoga
with a partner can increase the intimacy of your bond
and deepen your understanding of one another.

key benefits

▶ Builds your sense of control over your body

▶ Increases awareness of both self and partner

▶ Encourages deep intimacy

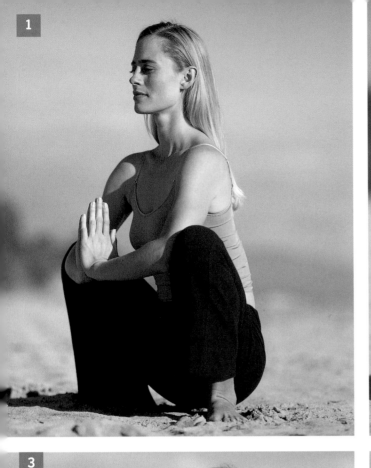

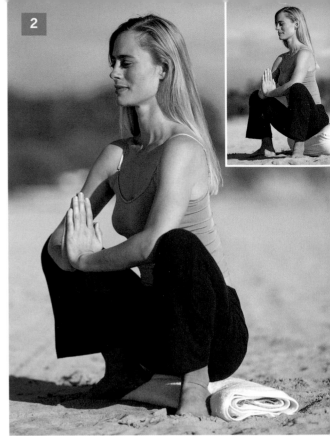

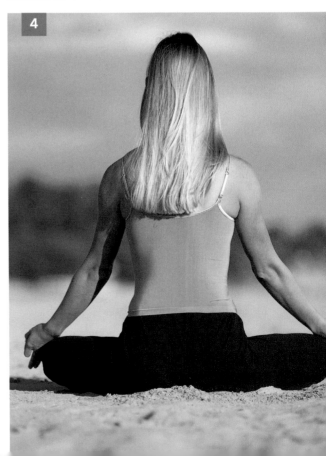

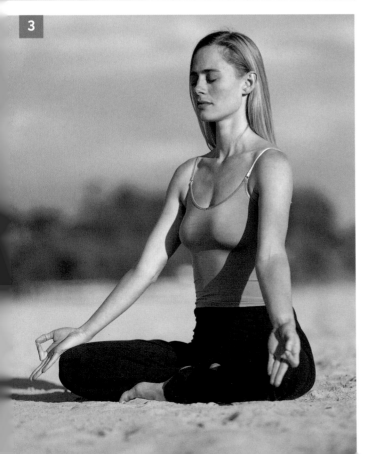

find your centre

These poses are designed to accentuate awareness of body, breath and gravity – leaving you feeling grounded and in sync with yourself and the world.

1 squat

Stand with your feet slightly turned out about shoulder-width apart; bring your palms together in front of your heart and inhale. Bending your knees, exhale as you lower your hips down into a squat. Then bring your elbows inside your legs; gently press them out against your knees and lift your chest as upright as possible. If you feel discomfort in your knees, release. Otherwise, hold for ten breaths, then stand.

2 supported squat

If your heels rise when you sink into Squat, try placing a folded towel or blanket under your heels for support. If Squat feels more challenging than you can enjoy, if you would like to try a longer hold, or if you feel any discomfort in your knees, squat on something higher, such as a bolster (see inset photo), a couple of firm pillows or a low stool. Hold for ten breaths, then stand.

3 root lock

Sitting in a comfortable cross-legged position, squeeze and lift the soft floor of your pelvis (the pubococcygeus, a muscle that runs from the pubic bone to the tailbone). Hold this contraction for as long as you comfortably can, or practise rounds of squeezing and releasing. For added intensity, practise this in the Squat position and try to maintain the contraction as you stand up from Squat.

4 microcosmic orbit

Sitting comfortably, practise the Full Yogic Breath (described at right), focusing on your breathing. As you inhale slowly and deeply, visualise light or energy gathering at the base of your torso and rising to the crown of your head. Exhale slowly, envisioning the energy cascading back down from your crown. Repeat for a few minutes. You may also use this visualisation in any other pose or as a seated meditation.

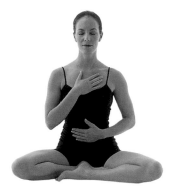

Full Yogic Breath

Deergha swaasam, the Full Yogic Breath, helps to calm your mind and refresh your body. Because you use the full capacity of your lungs, this breathing practice dramatically increases your oxygen intake. Inhale through your nostrils from the abdomen upwards, expanding your abdomen and ribcage, then lifting your collarbones. As you exhale, first relax your collarbones, then your ribcage and finally your abdomen. To feel the motion of your breath, place one hand on your chest and the other on your abdomen.

two become one

When two people move together in a shared yoga pose, both develop a unique awareness of each body in relation to the other and of how to work together to hold a safe and pleasurable position.

1 ecstatic arch

Stand toe-to-toe and grasp each other's wrists. In unison, inhale as you lift your chests. Exhale as you lean back slowly, lifting and arching your upper backs, necks and heads until you both have your arms straight; do not drop your heads back. Feel the rising momentum and the mutual support. Hold for several breaths, then together pull up to standing.

2 wide warriors

Stand with your feet about 90 to 120 cm apart, back-to-back with your partner. Turn your right (front) foot out 90 degrees and your left (back) foot slightly left, keeping your heels in line. Hold your arms parallel to the ground, palms down, and look right as you inhale. Ask your partner to mirror these instructions on his left side. Keeping your spine vertical, exhale as you bend your forward knee and bring it over your heel; try to lower your thigh parallel with the ground. Hold for 4–10 breaths. Release and repeat on the other side.

3 hands to hearts

Stand face-to-face with your partner (or try this sitting or lying down). Place your right hand over your partner's heart and your left hand on his lower back; ask him to do the same for you. Gaze into each other's eyes and practise the Microcosmic Orbit (see pose 4, page 105 ◄), feeling the depth of your union. Hold as long as you remain comfortable; extended practice can be an intense form of meditation.

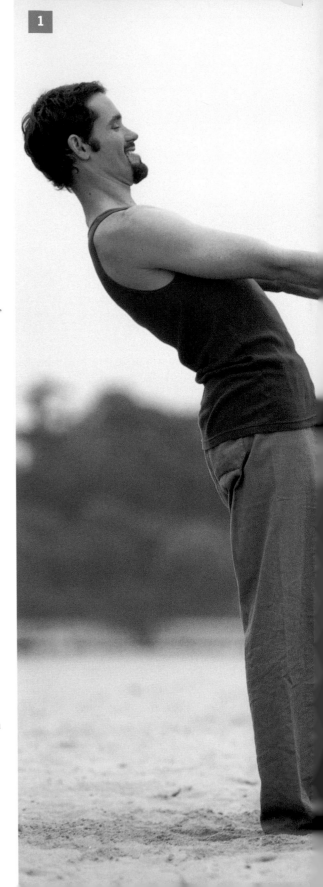

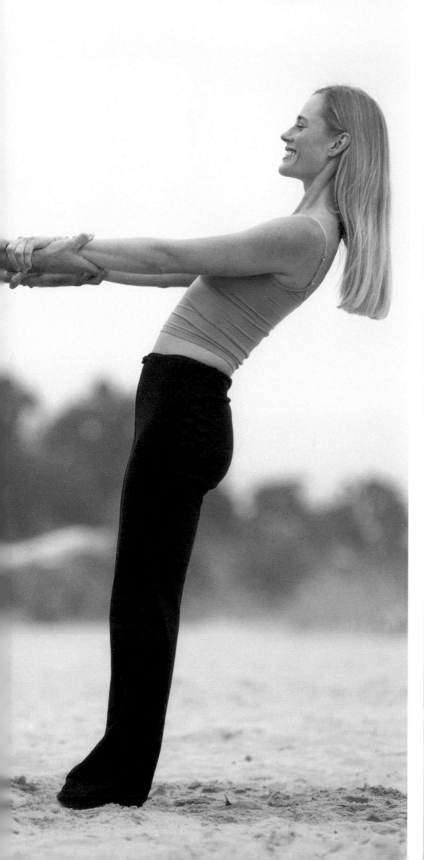

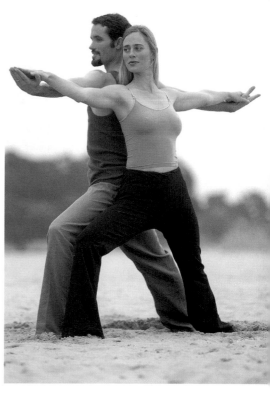

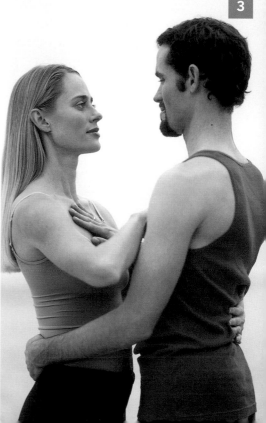

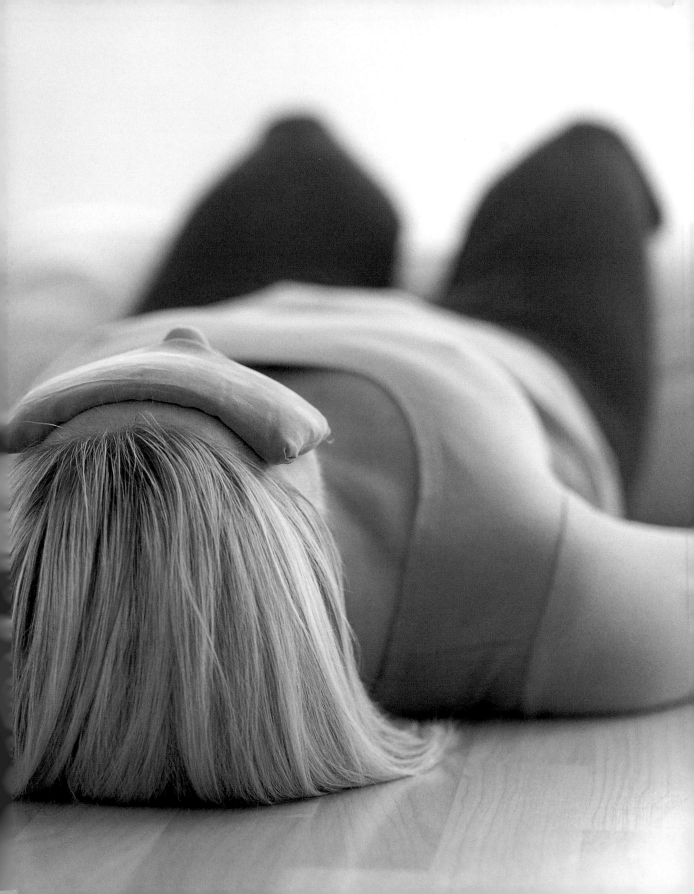

bliss

The ability to relax is a skill, and as with any skill, proficiency increases with practice. Deep relaxation is a form of meditation and visualisation that is traditionally performed at the end of a yoga session. Including it in your routine allows the benefits of the poses you've practised to permeate and restore you.

key benefits

▶ Helps you achieve profound relaxation

▶ Increases feeling of wellbeing

▶ Restores body and soul

go within

Amazing things happen when you practise deep relaxation. Meditation and visualisation exercises can help you feel comforted, calm – even blissful.

Bliss Out
- The aroma of lavender is known for its relaxing and balancing qualities. Try adding 2–3 drops of lavender essential oil to a bath to create a blissfully tranquil soak, or combine lavender with rose, patchouli, jasmine or ylang-ylang essential oil in a diffuser or a pillow spray.
- During deep relaxation practice, your body will cool down, so you might want to cover yourself with a blanket. For added comfort, place a rolled towel under your neck.

1 squeeze and scan

Traditionally, yoga practice ends with a period of relaxation and meditation: lie on your back, either flat or, for more comfort, with a pillow or bolster beneath your knees and an eye pillow over your eyes. Inhale, then hold your breath, making fists as you lift your arms several centimetres; contract and squeeze them for a few seconds, then exhale, dropping them. Repeat with your legs and feet. Inhale deeply and puff out your belly; hold, then release. Inhale deeply and expand your chest; hold, then release. Gently rock your head from side to side a few times. Scrunch up your face tightly; then stretch it out by sticking out your tongue and rolling your eyes upwards.

Relax and mentally scan your body slowly and thoroughly, gradually moving your awareness from your toes to your head. Spend a few moments focusing on each part of your body. If you sense areas of muscular tension or energy blockage, visualise those places softening and relaxing. You might imagine a wave of warm light slowly rising through your body, creating a perfect state of physical ease. When you feel completely relaxed, mentally observe your body at ease.

2 witness and rise

Continue lying on your back. Observe your breath and its natural flow. If you notice your mind has wandered, simply return your focus to your breath. After a minute or so, draw your awareness to your thoughts and witness them without judgement as they come and go for a few minutes. Become aware of inner calmness or even bliss.

Spend about five minutes deepening your breath, enjoying the focused calm you have created, then roll over onto your right side, cradling your right arm beneath your head, and bending your knees and bringing them towards your chest. When you feel ready to sit up, rise slowly. Let your body and thoughts remain in a state of calm.

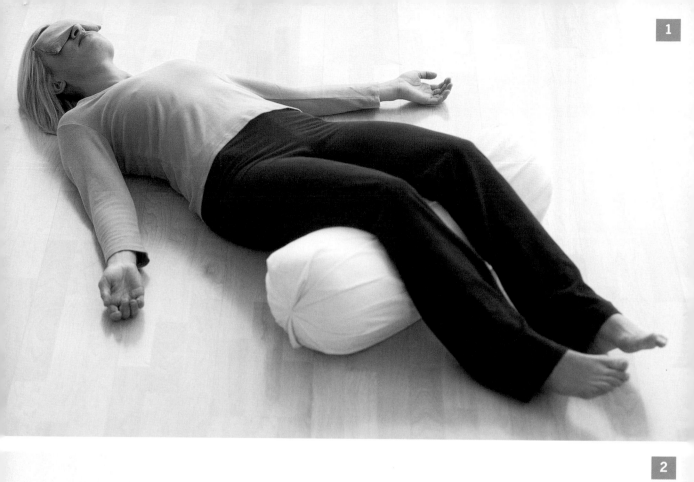

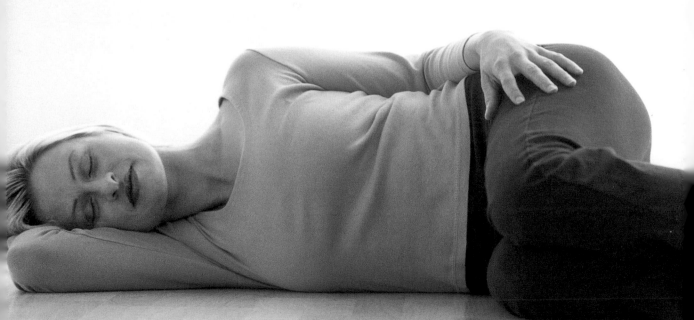

index

acknowledgements

We wish to thank the following people for their generous assistance in producing this book: Joanna Brown, Jane Burley and Tracey Edwards from The Body Shop International; Peter Cieply, managing editor, and Madhuri Fiona Flynn, consulting editor, for the hardback edition; Lisa Milestone and Jackie Mancuso for design assistance; Gail Nelson-Bonebrake and Kate Washington for copyediting; Cynthia Rubin, Tom Hassett, Renée Myers and Elissa Rabellino for proofreading; Ken DellaPenta for indexing; Virginia McLean for research; make-up artist France Dushane; photo assistant Marks Moore; models Scott Blossom, Helen Demuth, Chandra Easton, Vajra Farnsworth, Kristie Dahlia Home, Joan Jurado-Blanco, Athena Pappas, Justine Roddick, Maiya Roddick-Fuller, Michael Schindele, Laura Schlieske, Angella Sprauve, Brent Thomas, Lea Watkins, Amy Wood and Liz Yee; San Francisco City Lights for clothing.